Why Walk?

Discover the Transformative Power of an Intentional Walking Practice

Joyce Shulman

Kibo Press

Front cover design by Kamelija Gievska & Nina Dec
Front cover photo by Andy Stark

ISBN: 978-1-7342576-2-5

First printing edition 2023.

Kibo Press
99 Highview Drive
Sag Harbor, NY 11963

www.joyceshulman.com

Introduction

My son was born on a cold January night. What started as a typical labor became an emergency c-section complete with a plummeting heart rate (his), a missed epidural (mine), and a flurry of commotion when they thought they left a sponge someplace it wasn't supposed to be.

I recall several long, long minutes while the nurses counted, and recounted, until Bernadette, the labor and delivery nurse who had been by my side since labor began hours before, retrieved the wayward sponge from the floor.

"I've got it!" she cried.

The doctors put me back together and handed me my newborn son.

We were released from the hospital four days later and I returned home battered, postpartum, and totally freaked out.

Other than a couple of doctors' appointments and one slightly traumatic trip with my mother to buy nursing bras, I didn't leave the house for a month. And my husband and I? We were co-parenting, but not connecting.

Then, one morning, we woke up to bright, brilliant sunshine, a rarity in New York in February. We bundled the baby up, placed him gingerly in the stroller, and went for a walk around our neighborhood.

I can still feel the handle of the stroller and the sun on my face, and I can picture the hideous yellow maternity jacket that was still the only thing that fit.

And I vividly recall looking at my husband and saying, *"We can do this."*

That was the turning point.

That wasn't the first time that walking saved me, nor was it the last.

In college, I lost more than 30 pounds walking. On a hiking trip in British Columbia, I developed the idea that would become our first truly successful business. And during the hundreds of hours I've spent walking with friends, we have talked about everything – and I mean everything – kids, work, politics, relationships, hopes, dreams, menopause, and, well, *everything*.

I have solved more problems, shaken off more stress, generated more ideas, and lost more weight walking than through any other practice or habit. It has kept me sane, fit, and healthy.

I am not alone.

Many of history's greatest thinkers, innovators, creators, and world changers – from Aristotle to Beethoven, from Henry David Thoreau to Steven Jobs, from Darwin to Socrates and the dozens of people you will meet in the coming pages – understood the power of walking. Each had a regular, consistent, and lifelong walking practice.

All understood, instinctively, what research has begun to reveal: just how powerful, impactful, and downright transformative the simple act of a regular walking practice can be. It can reduce your risk of high-blood pressure, diabetes, dementia, and several types of cancer. It can fuel your creativity, improve your decision-making, build your executive function, and literally make your brain bigger.

Walking is a powerful tool to combat depression, reduce stress and anxiety, boost your mood, and enable you to tap into a powerful sense of awe. It can bring people and communities together.

All this from the simple act of lacing up your sneakers and walking at the door?

Yup, all this. And lots more. More happiness. More energy. More vitality. More life worth living.

Sounds too good to be true? I know.

Are We Sure? The Story of A Time-Traveling Dietician

Years ago, I watched a hilarious video titled *This is Why Eating is Hard*. The video opens with a woman cooking breakfast for her thickly-mustached husband. The year is 1979. With her ironed-straight hair, pea-green kitchen, and groovy pants, she lays a plate of fried eggs, toast, and steak on the table. Before her husband takes his first bite, a time-traveling dietitian appears from the future to warn the man not to eat the cholesterol-laden eggs, cautioning that "eating just one egg can dramatically increase your chance of heart attack." The wife, grateful for the advice, grabs the offending eggs from the table as the dietitian disappears.

Moments later, the dietitian returns from the slightly more recent past. "Wait," he cries, "we were wrong about the eggs. It is the egg yolks that are bad, the whites are fine." The wife, relieved, though a bit confused, thanks the dietitian who disappears again, only to return in a flash from the even more recent past. "Turns out we don't even know exactly what cholesterol is and the eggs are probably fine for you. But the steak," he yells, "no steak." It's the red meat that causes heart attacks, he cautions. In a flash, the dietitian leaves once again only to return to warn of the dangers of bread. "Man was not meant to eat bread," he yells.

By the final visit, both husband and wife have lost all confidence in the time-traveling dietitian and his constantly conflicting warnings.

The video drives home the contradictions inherent in decades of evolving advice about health, wellness, and fitness. Add a multi-billion dollar industry set on convincing us that wellness and weight loss can be easily obtained by buying this book, drinking this potion, or joining this gym, and it is no wonder that many of us are confused, discouraged, and skeptical.

Despite the many twists and turns, research continues to evolve and improve. We have never known more about what it takes to be fit and well than we do now. And yet, as a society, we are becoming less fit and less well.

Obesity – and the myriad of health risks associated with carrying more than 20% excess weight – continues to rise at astounding rates. According to the Centers for Disease Control and Prevention (CDC), between 2000 and 2018, the prevalence of obesity increased from 30.5% to 42.4%: a rise of more than 40% in fewer than 10 years. And the incidence of related, preventable diseases, such as heart disease, stroke, type 2 diabetes, and several types of cancer, continues to rise right along with it.

It is not just our physical bodies that are suffering – mentally and emotionally we are suffering as well, as levels of burn-out continue to increase as our attention spans continue to decrease. And last, but certainly not least, we are becoming unhappier. Research over the past several decades has shown that levels of depression, anxiety, and suicide continue to rise with one report revealing that diagnoses of major depression rose 33% between 2013 and 2018 – a figure most experts agree would be materially higher if it were to include undiagnosed depression.

Why? Of course, the causes are complicated. We are living with too much isolation. We are eating too much sugar. We are addicted to our devices. We are sitting too much. We live amidst ongoing racial injustice, political upheaval, and an always-on, mostly negative news cycle. And more.

How do we begin to course correct? Is there one practice, one habit, one routine, one behavior that has the power to impact pretty much all that is wrong?

Walking.

Yes, I know that is a very bold claim. And no, a regular walking practice will not instantly fix all of society's ills. It will not miraculously cure obesity, heart disease, dementia, depression, and burnout. It will not make every lonely person feel the power of connection. It will not magically cure all depression and prevent every suicide. It will not bring every community together or right every social injustice.

But it can help. A lot.

In the coming pages, we will delve into the research, meet dozens of people whose lives have been transformed by their walking practice, and explore practical tips and advice on how you can reap the powerful benefits of an intentional walking practice.

The time-traveling dietician put a hilarious point on the fact that advice about nutrition seems to change overnight, often reversing itself entirely. Eggs, good or bad? Toast, mana or poison? Meat, yes or no? Though the research continues to improve and evolve, there is a whole lot of conflicting information and advice about what, when, and how to eat.

But the benefits of walking?

Thousands of years of practice and hundreds of years of research has consistently taught us that Hippocrates, the father of modern medicine, was right when he declared "walking is man's best medicine."

The Myth of the 10,000 Steps and Power of Intentional Walks

Anyone who watches television, reads magazines, or scrolls social media could reasonably assume that the key to health, happiness, and longevity is taking 10,000 steps each day. It is typically what it takes to close the rings on your smartwatch and lets you check the box of a job well done on your to-do list.

Where did that 10,000 step-goal come from? Marketing, not medicine. In the 1960s, a Japanese company created a pedometer they named *Manpo-kei*, which translates to "10,000 steps meter." They marketed that device on the premise that 10,000 steps a day was the ideal number for health and wellness. Somehow, that idea spread and stuck.

Is it true? Is 10,000 daily steps the magic number?

We will discover that it doesn't look that way.

Now, don't get me wrong, more movement is good. Many of us – dare I say most of us – sit too much and move too little. Finding ways to get more physical activity into our days is likely to be good for us. So go ahead, park your car at the far end of the parking lot, get off the bus two stops early, or get a treadmill desk so you can walk while you work.

But there are far greater benefits to be gained from an intentional walking practice.

Our goal is not simply more life – though more life is awesome. Yet the true goal is strengthening our hearts, improving our moods, managing our stress, fueling our creativity, and fostering real connections with others. Being happier. Living a fuller, better, richer life. Longer, sure, but not just longer, better. An intentional walking practice can deliver benefits far beyond those gained by sneaking more steps into your day.

What's an "Intentional Walk"?

What do I mean by an "intentional walk"?

I define an intentional walk as taking some measure of time – be it fifteen minutes or fifty minutes – to step away from your computer, work, laundry, dishes, kids and social media. Sure, you can take company ... a dog, a friend, or a stroller. You can walk on a trail, a sidewalk, or around the mall. You can head out at the crack of dawn, during your lunch break, in the late afternoon, or after dinner. It is the intention that matters: *"I am going to go for a walk."*

As we will explore in greater depth and detail, taking an intentional walk, especially one at a brisk pace, provides the opportunity to raise your heart rate for a period of time, which is essential to improving your cardiovascular health and to reaping a myriad of powerful benefits for your body – from your bones to your brain.

Taking an intentional walk also delivers a host of benefits for your mind and your mood. It gives you the chance to lose yourself in thought or music or conversation and gives your brain the chance to rest and recharge. There is compelling evidence that it can boost your mood, combat depression, improve your concentration, sharpen your decision-making, and fuel your creativity.

And walking together? Magic. As we will discover, conversations had while walking have a uniquely intimate texture as they flow from topic to topic – the kind of conversations that forge the meaningful connections that we, as human beings, crave. It's the reason why women who regularly walk together are less likely to be lonely.

So go ahead, strive to increase your overall level of physical activity by increasing your daily step count. That's awesome. Go ahead and park at the far side of the parking lot, take the stairs rather than the escalator, and get off the bus two stops early. All of these choices will add physical activity to your day and contribute to your well-being.

But while adding more steps to your day can be valuable, intentional walks deliver so much more. Not just more life, but more joy and more happiness. And, as the philosopher Aristotle, famous for his practice of walking while he thought and while he taught (and who, not incidentally, lived to 62 at a time when the average life expectancy was about 32), reminds us, "Happiness is the meaning and the purpose of life, the whole aim and end of human existence."

What's To Come

This book has three parts. Part I explores the *why*. We will dig deep into research and stories that show how a regular walking practice unlocks tremendous reserves of potential and gives you the time to realize that potential. We will discover that walking is truly transformative for your mind, your mood, and your body.

In Part II, we get tactical. What to wear. When to walk. How fast, how slow, how often. What does the research teach us about exactly how much walking does it take to make an impact? We will discover that all walking is good, but walking in alignment, at particular times, and in particular ways can be even better.

Finally, in Part III, we'll discover how walking with other people can help forge the kind of meaningful connections that are key to a happy, fulfilling, productive, and long life. We will meet a walking school bus, a young Black man who has transformed communities by discovering the "walk sound" when neighbors walk together, a therapist who walks with his teenage clients, and we will explore the science behind why walking together is so powerful.

This book has been five years in the making because every time I think I've managed to explore and address every benefit of walking, I discover a new study or hear a new story that causes me to wonder if I have shared every benefit, every study, every tip, and every tactic about the myriad of benefits and perspectives of walking.

At some point, I had to say enough. I had to stop right where I was. I had to accept that I could not – and can not – share every benefit, direct you to every relevant study, and tell every story. Otherwise, I'd still be researching and writing and this book would never land in your hands.

And what was the goal really? The goal is to amaze you with the vast scope of benefits, share fascinating research and inspire you to lace up your sneakers and get moving. Because I believe – I know – that this one simple practice can change your life, change your family's life, and, ultimately, change the world.

Ready? Great, let's get going.

Oh, wait. One more thing before we dig in. I am not a doctor, a physical therapist, nor a scientist. What I am is a student of the connection between walking and the mind, mood, and body. During the course of researching and writing this book, I had the honor to interview hundreds of experts in their fields, read countless research papers, and interview thousands of people about the how, why, and benefits of walking. Any errors – and there are likely to be a few – are entirely my own. I include every study I reference in the appendix, and if there is a particular topic that interests you, I encourage you to consider this book a jumping off point and dig deeper.

Okay, now we're ready. Let's go.

Part I: The Benefits of Walking for Your Mind, Mood, and Body

Walking and Your Mind

"All truly great thoughts are conceived while walking."
Friedrich Nietzsche

It was almost two decades ago when we were contemplating adding a second child to our family and to our small two-bedroom house. A house that had been built out of what seemed like cardboard as a summer retreat, never intended to be a full-time home for a family of four. When the wind blew hard, the walls shook, and when the rain fell steadily outside, it also fell in the middle of the living room. Sure, we could have put both kids – the toddler and the baby – in a bedroom together, but it was tiny, and one was a boy and one was a girl so really, how long was that going to work?

We decided to build an addition over the garage – a master bedroom and bathroom, freeing up our current room for the baby and leaving our young son in the room he had already grown attached to. We borrowed what we could, and that got us a shell of a room that was intended to house a bedroom, bathroom, and closet. We were stuck with an open square of space with plywood on the floor and no sheetrock on the walls. How to configure it? We had no money to hire an architect and, as I often do, I thought *"how hard can it be?"* Yet I couldn't solve the puzzle.

I called Margo. "Can you come over?" I asked her. "I need your brain on something."

Margo is an immensely talented jewelry designer, but more than that, she is a creative spirit who had recently renovated her own home. I hoped she could help.

She arrived an hour later, walked once around the raw space, careful to step over the pile of lumber that still sat in the middle of the floor. "Okay," she said, "this is easy. The bathroom goes here," she pointed, "and the closet here. You'll need about this much space between them and oh," she added, "it would be awesome if you added some glass high up on the wall between the bedroom and the bathroom, because that will let in all the morning light. Give me a piece of paper and I'll sketch it out for you."

It took her no more than two minutes to solve something I'd been staring at for weeks and in that moment, I thought, *"her brain works very differently than mine."* Give me a dozen law cases to synthesize or a complex situation to untangle, challenge me to identify a business's fundamental flaw or big opportunity and I will deliver. Ask me to figure out how to configure 500 square feet and I was lost.

Over the years I've gotten better, and a decade later when we were designing our new home, I was the one who figured out the layout for the new second floor: three bedrooms, three closets, two bathrooms. We've been living in what I sketched on a scrap of paper for years and it's been perfect.

Those experiences taught me two things. I realized that different people's brains work differently. Margo sees things I never will. But I also realized that even I can learn to see things through a different lens and in a different way. My brain, my talents, my cognitive abilities are not fixed – they are flexible and, with exercise and practice, can continue to grow and develop.

Our brains are the essence of life and self. How we think, what we feel, where we go, and the choices we make. Our well-being is reflective of how clearly our minds function, how creatively we can solve life's inevitable challenges, how we continue to learn new things and how we maintain our cognitive abilities as we age.

At some point, many of us begin to lose our ability to grasp the names of people we know. I have felt it happen to me from time to time and witnessed the slow but steady decline as my dad, who never forgot the name of a single one of his students, would struggle to recall the name of a niece or nephew. It is one of life's biggest injustices: for many, our minds give out before our bodies.

To maximize the quality of our lives, we must do what we can to protect and improve the functioning of our minds. Being able to think more clearly, create more effectively, understand more deeply, and pay attention more closely enables us to live more fully.

What does this have to do with exercise in general and walking in particular? Everything. Now, most of what you'll find about the power of physical activity focuses on how it affects our bodies. *Lose weight! Get stronger! Improve your heart health! Live longer!* And, while those are valuable, important goals, the most important contribution exercise makes is to our minds, because without them, what good are stronger abs or a longer life?

Over the coming pages, we'll explore the many ways a regular, intentional walking practice will impact our minds. We will:

- Take a dive into the brain's white matter and gray matter;
- Hear about the day I took my executive function for a walk;
- Be reminded of the importance of sleep;
- Contemplate all of the possible uses for a pillow;
- Discover that walking might be better than dancing to improve memory;
- Explore the beauty of a weighty hippocampus;
- Learn how walking helps untangle the thoughts of one of the world's most creative people; and
- Conclude that Nietzsche was right when he famously observed that "all truly great thoughts are conceived while walking."

Who Knew?

Aristotle knew. More than 2,000 years after his death, the Ancient Greek philosopher and scientist's writings and teachings remain vibrant, important, and instructive. He wrote and spoke on morality and public speaking, poetry and politics, and, ultimately, happiness and the meaning of life. Balanced with reality and responsibility, Aristotle understood that happiness was not a state or a destination, but rather an active practice.

Aristotle was famous for his walking. He walked while he taught. He walked while he thought. He walked while he collaborated with his teacher and friend Plato. By most accounts, he produced his greatest insights and taught his most valuable lessons while walking.

Thousands of years later, Steve Jobs, considered one of the most demanding and brilliant innovators of our time, made walking a regular part of his practice. He was frequently spotted walking the Apple campus, and often held meetings – especially meetings where creativity was key – while walking. Jobs' habit of walking barefoot around the Apple campus has become the stuff of Silicon Valley lore.

Jobs and Aristotle were not alone. Other legendary innovators, creators, and thinkers who made walking a meaningful part of their personal and professional practice include Charles Darwin, Benjamin Franklin, Ludwig van Beethoven, Ralph Waldo Emerson, Charles Dickens, and countless others.

Science is catching up with what these innovators instinctively knew was right and over the past few decades, neuroscience has revealed a great deal about how walking helps us think and perform better.

Not only does walking help our brains perform better, but over time a regular walking practice can cause positive changes to our brain's actual structure, by strengthening the scaffolding, encouraging the formation of neurons, and thus building stronger, bigger brains.

Walking Makes Your Brain More Plastic (and that's a good thing)

Sometime last year, I was listening to an interview with one of the world's leading neurologists. I wish I could remember his name, but sadly, I can't. In his late 70s at the time of the interview, he had begun his medical career in the 1960s, nearly two years before the MRI was invented and long before the explosion of insights into how the brain works.

As the doctor described it, when he launched his career, the human brain was something of a black box. Doctors and neuroscientists had only a rudimentary understanding of what went on when we thought thoughts, experienced emotions, or strove to move mountains.

Bit by bit, they began unlocking that black box, gaining insights into how our brains work, and discovering ways we can best care for that most complicated and incredible human organ. While we have a long, long way to go to fully understand its mysteries, we know enough to do a better job taking care of our brain.

One of the biggest changes in how the adult brain is viewed is the concept of neural plasticity. As recently as 20 years ago, the generally accepted thinking – no pun intended – was that children's brains were malleable and able to generate new neurons and form new connections, but once you reached adulthood, your brain became largely fixed. You can't teach an old dog new tricks, right?

I found that concept very discouraging. I hated the idea that my brain power – my ability to learn, grow, and develop – was fixed and limited. Fortunately, more sophisticated research has revealed this is not true. Adult brains do continue to generate new neurons and form new pathways, albeit just at a slower rate than children. This process, called neurogenesis, continues throughout our lives.

Once that discovery was made, researchers began to explore what we can do to improve the function of our brains in the short term and maintain their best possible function as we age.

Among the most powerful steps we can take to help our brains function at their very best, for the longest time possible? Walking.

Walking Helps the Physical Structure of our Brains

Let's consider our brain's physical structure. On average, a human brain weighs about three pounds, consumes 20% of our oxygen and calories, and is incapable of feeling physical pain. It is command central, managing both our conscious and unconscious thoughts, movements, and emotions.

Yet we rarely give them a second thought – most of us spend more time thinking about the size of our hips, the wrinkles around our eyes, or what we are going to have for dinner.

Perhaps it is because our brain seems far too mysterious to contemplate or comprehend. I get that. How do you even begin to understand a weirdly shaped orb we carry around with us in our heads that scientists estimate can process billions of calculations per second? Billions.

Add to that the fact that, despite tremendous gains in recent years, the workings of our brain remain shrouded in mystery. The brain's complexity is mind boggling. The ability to process ideas, connect concepts, store memories, smell, taste, experience love, sneeze, all while keeping a heart beating, lungs breathing, and sometimes orchestrating the lifting of a coffee cup to a mouth? It's not an overstatement to declare your brain miraculous.

Not to terribly oversimplify it, but brains are composed of two different types of stuff – well, more than two really, but for now, let's focus on white matter and gray matter.

Bigger is Better: Walking Builds Gray Matter

Gray matter encompasses the approximately 86 billion neurons that enable us to do most of the things that we typically associate with our brains – it is generally responsible for our thoughts, emotions, memories, and movement. Despite the many remaining mysteries of the brain, scientists are in agreement that gray matter matters, that having more of it is generally better and may be linked with higher intelligence. It is most often studied, discussed, and considered when researchers consider the impacts of injury and aging.

One of the brain's critical structures is the hippocampus. Small, seahorse shaped, and located deep in the temporal lobe, the hippocampus is critical for learning, memory, and spatial navigation. Recent studies suggest that the hippocampus also plays a role in how we process and regulate our emotions; perhaps because our memories play a role in our emotions. Or perhaps not. Like I said, the workings of our brains remain pretty mysterious.

While there is variation as to when our brain's gray matter begins to deteriorate and the exact rate of decline varies by individual, the research is unequivocal: beginning somewhere around 50, the volume of our gray matter starts to decline. Specifically with respect to the all-important hippocampus, studies have shown that its volume typically decreases by 1% to 2% each year.

Not great.

Are there things we can do to positively impact the volume and health of our brain's gray matter? I suppose, at this point, it won't surprise you to discover that exercise – including walking – can have an impact. How much of an impact? Research has shown that a regular walking program can reverse the deterioration of your brain's gray matter, increase the volume of your hippocampus and literally makes your brain bigger.

In one compelling study, researchers divided 120 older adults into two groups and assigned each a different year-long exercise program:

- Group One walked 40 minutes three times each week; and
- Group Two engaged in an integrated, professionally-guided exercise program that included stretching, strengthening, balance, and yoga.

MRI imaging was used to compare the hippocampus volumes of each group before and after the program.

The walking group showed about a 2% *increase* in the volume of their hippocampus, while the stretching/resistance training group showed a 1.4% *decrease*.

The researchers concluded: "In sum, we found that the hippocampus remains plastic in late adulthood and that one year of aerobic exercise was sufficient for enhancing volume. Increased hippocampal volume translates to improved memory function."

Yup, more walking means a bigger brain.

Stronger Scaffolding: Walking Builds More Efficient White Matter

White matter is the scaffolding, the infrastructure, the superhighway of our brains. It is the wiring (of course, it's not literal wiring) that connects the brain's various regions, enabling us to process and perform.

When our brain's white matter begins to deteriorate, so do we.

Historically, most studies have focused on the brain's gray matter, and as we've discussed, exercise in general, and walking in particular, is incredibly beneficial for gray matter. But what about the white matter? Can walking help protect and even restore the brain's white matter? Preliminary research suggests that it can.

A study from Colorado State University sought to evaluate the impact of three different types of programs on the brain health of more than 240 generally healthy, but sedentary, older adults. First, the subjects' brains were scanned using a sophisticated form of MRI analysis that enabled the researchers to evaluate the condition of the white matter. Once that baseline was established, the participants were divided into three groups:

- Group One began a supervised stretching and balance exercise program;
- Group Two met three times a week to walk together; and
- Group Three participated in three weekly dance classes where they learned and practiced coordinated choreography.

After six months, the subjects returned to the lab to have their fitness evaluated and their brains rescanned.

Not surprisingly, the dancers and the walkers showed improvement in their aerobic fitness. But what about their brains? Both groups showed improvement in their brains' white matter – notably in those regions associated with memory and executive function. But the results revealed a surprise.

The researchers had hypothesized that the dance group would show the greatest improvement because those participants were simultaneously exercising, learning, and memorizing. But this hypothesis proved to be wrong: The walking group showed greater improvement in the white matter of their brains than the dancing group, despite the fact that the dancing group had the collective benefit of physical movement and aerobic conditioning, combined with the benefits of learning and memorizing choreographed dances.

The researchers cautioned that the study employed a relatively new type of analysis to evaluate the impact of different types of exercise on the plasticity of the white matter of the brain. Nevertheless, the study strongly suggests that not only is exercise good for your brain, but a regular walking practice may be more protective and beneficial to the brain's white matter than stretching, balance exercises, or dance classes.

What About How Our Brain Functions?

Okay. So walking can help support the physical structure of our brains, but what about improvements in how our brains actually function? Can walking help us think more clearly? Process more quickly? Remember more accurately? Love more deeply?

As we age, how can we maintain the highest possible brain function for the longest possible time?

Against the backdrop of the structural improvements, let's explore the powerful mental enhancements elicited by a regular walking practice.

I Wonder Where that Trail Goes: Walking and Executive Function

Last week, I took my executive function for a walk.

I tend to walk the same trails over and over. There's the 2.2 mile dirt road that starts at the back of the tiny 9-hole golf course and ends at the bay. There's the 2.8 mile loop that starts at the other side of that golf course, runs along the bay, and comes back up that same dirt road. There's the two-mile parking lot that runs alongside a different bay beach. I walk one of these three trails 90% of the time.

But last week, I did something different. I was on my beloved back-of-the-golf-course walk when I noticed a trail that intersected the dirt road and veered off to the north. Of course I've seen it before. I've walked this road hundreds, maybe thousands, of times, but that morning, I found myself staring at it, wondering where it went.

Feeling a spark of curiosity, I stepped onto it. "I'll just go for a few minutes and then I'll turn around," I thought. I had no idea where it went and I didn't want to get lost.

But I had a bit of time and the trail kept pulling me forward. After a few minutes, I noticed a blue trail marker on a tree. "Okay," I thought, "I'm on a marked trail, that's good." I kept going. After about ten minutes, I thought I saw a clearing beyond the trees in front of me. "A pond in the middle of the woods?" I wondered. Still curious, I continued walking toward it as my brain struggled to figure out where I was and where I was going.

As I got closer to the "pond," it occurred to me that I was still heading north and I realized that wasn't a pond at all – it was the bay. I had unknowingly made a loop. As I soldiered on, I connected with a trail off to my left, turned, and began to walk back to the golf course. It was a real life puzzle that I navigated as I went. There were a few moments when I had no idea where I was and felt a little tingle of fear. But as I put one foot in front of the other, I figured it out.

And in doing so, I took my executive function for a walk and found myself somewhere new and familiar all at the same time.

It seems to me that our "executive function" is misnamed. It has nothing to do with being an executive and everything to do with simply being able to function at our cognitive best.

Generally, executive function refers to our working memory, our self-control, and our ability to think flexibly. These three overarching elements manifest themselves in our ability to focus and pay attention, organize, plan and prioritize, control our emotions, and our behavior – essentially our overall cognitive function. People struggling with executive function may have difficulty prioritizing or completing tasks, following a sequence of steps, maintaining concentration, planning, managing their time, staying organized, or regulating their emotions. Yup, it is your overarching cognitive operating system.

Executive function is primarily governed by the area of your brain called the frontal lobe, which also houses our neural pathways and other brain networks. In other words, it's the way some parts of your brain communicate with other parts of your brain. Like with so, so many things, a regular walking practice has been shown to materially improve executive function.

In what they deemed the first study of its kind, a group of researchers in 2014 set out to explore whether a single bout of low-intensity exercise such as walking would have a positive impact on executive function. They noted that, as we've discussed, previous studies had shown that regular exercise can lead to positive structural changes of the brain and can reduce the risks of 44 age-related cognitive decline and neurological diseases, but that less research had been done on the effect of a single low-intensity exercise session on cognition and brain function.

25 college-aged individuals did merely 10-minutes of low-intensity exercise at a level of exertion comparable to walking. The researchers evaluated activation in their prefrontal cortex (the area of the brain that governs executive function) and tested their performance on a color-matching challenge that assesses executive function performance. The conclusion? A 10-minute bout of mild exercise resulted in a "significant" improvement in executive function.

What Can You Do With a Pillow: Walking and Creativity

Dr. Claudia K. Beeny is the founder of the House of Shine, a museum and community center in Dallas, Texas, designed to help people ages 5 to 95 unearth their talents and figure out how to use them to make the world a better and brighter place. Spend just five minutes with Claudia and you quickly discover that creativity is her love language. A fountain of fresh, fun ideas, she is widely recognized as an extraordinary creative thinker. "Claudia's superpower is ideation. Her steady flow of creative ideas would impress Walt Disney himself," says House of Shine COO, Colleen Monroe.

One key to Claudia's creativity? Walking, a practice she began as a teenager.

"Most school days, I walked from my high school to the gym and then home. Early on, it cultivated an awareness that walking was physically and mentally good for me. I loved the quiet, getting lost in my own thoughts, and noticing the same landmarks as they changed through the seasons."

Claudia continues her practice of walking the same route, alone and in silence. "In a world that is getting progressively noisier, carving out time to be alone, so that my mind can wander and my head can hear my heart, is something I get very excited about," she explains.

Claudia credits her walking practice with much of her creative output. "I'm confident that neither my dissertation, the blog I published daily for six years, the book I wrote, nor the House of Shine would have come to fruition if I did not walk regularly. Walking allows me to make valuable connections, recognize associations, and solve some of my toughest problems."

She is hardly alone. Author and philosopher Henry David Thoreau observed in his personal journal that, "the moment my legs begin to move my thoughts begin to flow" and philosopher Friedrich Nietzsche famously declared, "All truly great thoughts are conceived by walking."

But is it true? Is all of this anecdotal evidence that walking helps to fuel creativity true?

Science says it is.

Before we delve into the research that has demonstrated that Claudia's experience is not unique – and that Thoreau, Nietzche, and hundreds of other brilliant creatives were right – let's be sure we are on the same page with what we mean by creativity.

Tina Seelig, a Stanford professor and author of *Creativity Rules* – who "walks when she needs to think" – defines creativity as "applying your imagination to address a problem." Creativity embodies the ability to generate original ideas, view the world in a different way, connect ideas, identify patterns, or otherwise see things that are not, at first, obvious.

Over the years, social scientists have sought ways to test and measure creativity. Two such tests were employed by Stanford researchers Marily Oppezzo and Daniel L. Schwartz when they sought to understand the connection between walking and creativity.

The first was the Guilford's Alternate Use test, a deceptively simple exercise in which people are asked to identify as many different uses as possible for a common item within a fixed period of time. For instance, take five minutes to consider all of the potential uses for a pencil. Obviously, you can write with it. But what else could you do with it? If you have long hair, you can use it to hold your hair in a top knot. You could use it as a drumstick, or to punch holes in a piece of paper when you can't find a hole puncher. Perhaps you could use it as a weapon.

This is a fun exercise to try from time to time. Here are five possible prompts you can use but truly, the list is endless: Give yourself five minutes to come up with as many different uses can you think of for a:

- pillow;
- extension cord;
- button;
- nail clipper; or
- cotton swab.

The second test is Barron's Symbolic Equivalence Task where people are challenged to generate analogies. For instance, how many statements can you think of that are analogous to "a candle burning low" or "absence makes the heart grow fonder." The results are evaluated based on the number of analogies a person creates as well as the "quality" of those responses – essentially how analogous they are to the original statement.

In 2014, Oppezzo and Schwartz set out to test whether or not walking materially improved performance on these tests of creativity. Not surprising to anyone who has declared "I get my best ideas while walking," the answer was a resounding yes. Overall, walking improved people's creative output by 60%. Not only that, but the creative boost had a residual effect, powering people's creativity for hours after they returned from their walk and got back to work.

In 2019, another team of researchers from University of Graz in Austria again sought to explore the possible connection between movement and creativity. Over a five-day period, the researchers tracked the activity level of 79 adults and tested them on their ability to generate creative ideas. Once again, they discovered that those participants who walked more performed better on creative tests.

Here's how it works for me. I head out for a walk, usually for about 40 minutes, though an hour is better. As I begin walking, thoughts ping-pong around my head, bouncing among the email I was supposed to send but didn't, the five things still on my to-do list, the upcoming event I need to plan. I worry that I'm either underdressed for the walk and will be too cold, or overdressed and will be too warm. I fret about the work left undone, the dinner still to be prepared, and all of the other "more important" things that need to get done.

After ten minutes, my mind begins to settle as I find the rhythm of my walk. After about twenty minutes, ideas begin to flow. And then they don't stop.

About six months ago, I added a simple app to my watch. I hate to stop my walk, pull out my phone, and capture notes about all of the ideas that bubble up while I walk. But I also know that if I don't capture them fast, either while I am walking or immediately afterwards, they will disappear. Now, with the press of a big red button, I can quickly capture an audio note to myself, which the app will happily transcribe and email to me.

Walk. Imagine. Capture. Repeat.

There is nothing better to fire up your creativity than a walk.

Getting Unstuck: Walking and Problem Solving

Several months ago, I was wrestling with a particular work problem. While it seems simple in retrospect, it was thorny at the time: should we, or should we not, launch a series of virtual 5K events in addition to the monthly challenges we offer our customers? On the one hand, the community had been clamoring for them. On the other, the heart and soul of what we did were monthly walking challenges. It was during the Covid-19 pandemic and there were already hundreds of virtual races to be found. How could we give people something they couldn't get elsewhere? How could we make the experience transformative and special?

I did a lot of research and engaged in hours of discussion with my team. We surveyed our community for feedback. I had lots of information, lots of data, and lots of thoughts swirling around my head.

Lots of kindling, but no answer.

On a beautiful fall afternoon, I took all of that input with me on a three-mile walk. As I walked, I focused my attention on what exactly a weekend-long virtual event would be like. How could we make it unique and meaningful? What could we do to turn a one-hour 5k into a transformative weekend-long event? When my mind began to drift, which of course it did, I intentionally brought it back to a possible 5k weekend, asking myself, over and over, what happens next and how we can make it better?

In his book *Deep Work*, author Cal Newport dubbed this kind of practice "productive meditation" which he describes as taking "a period in which you're occupied physically but not mentally – walking, jogging, driving, showering – and focus your attention on a single well-defined professional problem."

It works. By the time I completed my walk, the plan had crystalized. I could see the entire 5k weekend playing out in my mind. The moment I got home, I spread three sheets of paper across my dining room table, one for each day, and sketched the blueprint that would become our first successful virtual event.

Productive walking. Walking with the intention of thinking through a particular issue. Training your mind to focus on one particular challenge.

Using your walk to solve one specific problem.

There's a caveat. This doesn't work all of the time. Just because you focus your mind and give your brain the opportunity to work at its very best does not guarantee that a solution will come to you. Problems are tricky things and solutions can be elusive. Some problems cannot be solved in one walk and some can't be solved in ten. But one thing is for sure: walking provides an excellent environment for you to do your very best problem solving.

Squirrel: Walking and Improved Focus

"I think I've ruined my brain." Eric and I were sitting outside on the deck late one fall afternoon.

"What do you mean?" he asked.

"It's so hard to hold a single thought, to focus on one thing. My brain is non-stop bouncing in a dozen different directions."

And then, like he was being paid to do it, a squirrel ran across the yard in front of us. Our dog, Moose, who had been laying quietly at my feet, bolted to action and sprinted across the yard.

"Squirrel," I said, following him with my eyes. No matter what Moose is doing, a squirrel cannot be ignored. It must be chased.

And that is how I find my mind these days, with squirrels presenting themselves in the form of emails, text messages, and social media notifications. Then there's the ability to seek the answer to any question that crosses my mind. *Hmm, I wonder what the weather will be today. Hmmm, I wonder if Michelle had her baby. Hmmm, I wonder if all dogs chase squirrels.* Give me a minute while I Google that ...

We've become so proficient at moving quickly from one thing to another that we've sacrificed our ability for deep and meaningful thought. Our reduced attention spans have been well documented in countless studies and bemoaned in countless articles.

I believe it. Before the advent of social media, back when I used to write first drafts by hand on a long legal pad rather than on the computer, I had a reliable three-hour attention span. I could dig deep into a project, focus intently, and do my best work for three hours after which my brain was tired and needed a break. But wow, the work I could produce during those three hours.

These days, getting to that place of genuine focus and deep work is far, far more challenging. There are all of the added responsibilities of life, all of the things that ring and ping and demand my attention, and the reality that I have trained my brain to crave the quick hit. Like most of us, I consume bite-sized bits of news and information, read most things for less than a minute, and scroll through social media feeds barely registering 90% of what I see. And I live my life on temptation island with my phone and computer offering up all measures of distraction.

Looking at my screen right now, there are eleven tabs open across the top and 26 icons just below the words I am typing. When I hit a block in my thinking it is oh so easy to simply click away or think, *maybe there's some research I haven't seen on this topic* or wonder *how was the engagement on that video I posted yesterday?*

We spend a lot of time staring at our phones and our computers. That is not new news. One study reported that we check our phones an average of 262 times each day. We live with a 24-hour news cycle and a constant barrage of stimulation. Our brains are constantly on, filtering, processing, and working. As a consequence of all of that input, we have sacrificed our ability to get lost in thought and let our minds do what they are uniquely qualified to do: to think interesting, creative thoughts and solve big, thorny problems.

Squirrel.

To better navigate our always-on world, we need tactics that allow our brains the chance to rest so our focus and concentration can be restored.

A walk can help. A raft of studies have looked at the impact of a single walk on our ability to concentrate, as well as how an ongoing walking practice can support enhanced concentration. While, with everything involving the brain, the "how" is complicated, the result is clear: walking helps you focus.

Oh, and by the way, according to our contemporary scholar, Google...

Not all dogs chase squirrels.

I Could Use a Few More Points: Walking and IQ

There are days when I would love just a few more points on my IQ, when I wish understanding came more quickly and connections came more easily. I guess I should keep walking, as studies have revealed a correlation between physical activity and cognitive horsepower.

In 2009, a group of Swedish researchers studied 1.2 million men enlisted for military service between 1950 and 1976. They sought to discover a possible connection between improved fitness and increased intellectual performance. The cohort included thousands and thousands of twins, which enabled the researchers to compare the impact of fitness on people who were genetically identical.

The study revealed "a clear positive association between cardiovascular fitness and cognitive performance in young adults," leading the researchers to conclude that "changes in physical achievement between ages 15 years and 18 years predicted cognitive performance at age 18 years." But the benefits didn't stop, as the researchers followed the men for several more years and discovered that "cardiovascular fitness during early adulthood predicted socioeconomic status and educational attainment later in life."

While the researchers pointed out that the study did not show direct causation – perhaps the smarter boys simply exercised more – the results demonstrated that "subjects with improved predicted cardiovascular fitness between 15 and 18 years of age exhibited significantly greater intelligence scores than subjects with decreased cardiovascular fitness."

Even among genetically identical twins.

Now, Where Did I Leave My Keys? Walking Improves Short-Term Memory.

When I was in law school, I claimed my favorite cubicle in the library. It was on the mezzanine floor, second from the wall on the right-hand side. I love my routines and had created a habit of sitting in that very space for long afternoons, struggling to encode 200 years of constitutional case law into my brain. Apparently, I was right and wrong. Habits are great to help us build our concentration muscle and keep us focused. But research suggests I would have been better off if, rather than sitting for hours at a time, I had integrated some walking into my study routine. Bonus points for walking backwards.

A study out of the University of California showed that even 10 minutes of light exercise, like walking, has a material impact on memory. Thirty-six volunteers in their early 20s – the exact same age I was while I was struggling to memorize the Federal Code of Civil Procedure – did 10 minutes of light exercise at an intensity comparable to walking while researchers observed their brain activity via MRI. The researchers then tested their memory and recall. On another day, the same group underwent the same memory tests without exercising. The results? Even a 10-minute bout of light exercise improved connectivity between the regions of the brain involved in memory and recall.

Apparently, rather than sitting for hours at a time struggling to decipher ancient legal briefs, the better plan would have been to walk, study, walk, study, walk, study. With the occasional cup of coffee, of course.

A final wacky note on walking and memory. Research has suggested that walking backwards – or even simply imagining yourself walking backwards – appears to boost your short-term memory. Dubbed the "mnemonic time-travel effect," this research, though preliminary, suggests that physically moving backwards somehow helps your mind travel backwards, thereby helping you recall recent memories. Can't find your keys? Try walking backwards!

My Dad is Still My Dad: Walking, Dementia, and Alzheimers

I grew up on one square acre in a classically suburban neighborhood about 40 minutes from New York City. My parents were "house people" – meaning our home was important to them and their most significant investment. We rarely went out for dinner, never went to the theater, and vacations were few and far between. But the house? We all loved the house. When I was a kid, I climbed every tree and dug under every rock. There was a boulder from which to launch the rope swing that hung from the oak tree in the backyard. Every fall, I would take a long pole and knock chestnuts from the pair of trees that lined the driveway and when the three huge poplar trees got sick and died, the family mourned.

And there was a well-worn path around the perimeter of the acre that delineated our property.

Each day, after my dad came home from work, he would change into shorts and a pair of converse sneakers and run slow laps around the house. This was years before "jogging" became popular. Though he was an accomplished sprinter in his youth, these laps around our yard were not about speed. They were about transitioning from the work-day to the evening. They were about getting the daily dose of exercise he knew his mind, mood, and body needed.

One time I visited my parents, where they now reside in Florida. At 92, my dad is still my dad. Though he occasionally loses the thread of a complicated television program and has been known to get distracted and leave the sink water running after he has finished shaving, he is as intuitive, smart, and conversational as always. And though his jogging days are long past, he still walks. Every day.

"You know," he said on that visit, "I'm convinced that walking and exercise have been key to longevity and to keeping my brain sharp." Yup, Dad, you're right – and you've been right all of these years.

As we age, our brains age right along with the rest of us and that aging can impact a variety of mental functions including our memory, language skills, problem-solving abilities, and more. Yup – those exact same executive function skills we mentioned earlier.

Depending on their severity and the way they affect one's life, these age-related declines cover a broad spectrum, from mild cognitive impairment to full-blown dementia.

And then there is Alzheimer's, a neurodegenerative disease that is the big daddy of cognitive decline. Though there is no cure and no magic bullet, by some estimates, a whopping 35 percent of cases of Alzheimer's disease and other forms of dementia could be delayed or prevented by lifestyle changes. High on that list of lifestyle interventions? Walking.

Several studies over the past two decades have identified a link between increased exercise – including a regular walking practice – and improved brain function. Walking has been shown not only to increase the efficiency of our brains, but also help stave off the mental declines often associated with aging.

In just one of many studies that have confirmed a link between physical activity and cognitive impairment, researchers looked at 3,903 adults aged 55 and older and tracked frequency of exercise (including walking) and their mental acuity over two years. The study concluded that, among the " moderate or high physical activity, compared with no physical activity, are independently associated with a lower risk of developing incident cognitive impairment after 2 years."

In another, a team of researchers sought to ascertain the efficacy of a six-month exercise program on the memory of women aged 70–80 who were suffering from mild cognitive impairment. Three groups were created and three exercise interventions were applied:

- Group One engaged in resistance training;
- Group Two walked outdoors; and
- Group Three participated in a combined stretching, flexibility, and balance program.

The researchers evaluated the subjects before and after the exercise program on two different types of memory typically associated with cognitive impairment: verbal memory and spatial memory. In a general sense, verbal memory relates to words or concepts while spatial memory relates to the position or location of objects or places.

In the verbal memory and learning test, the participants were given a list of 15 common words to read and then challenged to recall as many words from the list as possible immediately and again twenty minutes later.

In the spatial memory test, the participants were presented with a simple computerized game whereby they were challenged to remember the position of three dots that had appeared on a computer screen.

Here's what they discovered.

Group One – the women who participated in the outdoor walking program – remembered "significantly more" on the verbal memory test: 43.4% more than the stretching, flexibility, and balance group and almost 11% more than the resistance training group. The researchers concluded that twice-weekly aerobic training in the form of walking, over a six-month period resulted in "significantly improved verbal memory and learning" and "improved reaction times during the spatial memory test compared to the control group."

Research into how frequently, how intense, and how impactful regular exercise is on our mental functioning as we age continues to evolve, but the evidence is clear: regular exercise, including walking, can have a material impact on maintaining the functioning of our brains as we age.

How?

We began our discussion with the power of a regular walking practice to induce positive, structural changes to our brains and there is no doubt that increased gray matter and stronger white matter can improve the way our brains function.

But I don't think that's the entire answer as to how walking helps our brains work better. Indeed, how is it that a single walk can help restore focus, build concentration, and fuel creativity? Researchers aren't entirely sure and have posited several theories. Chances are, the mental refresh and benefits of walking result from a mix of them.

Perhaps it is the Power of our Default Mode Network

We often think of walking as an automatic skill that we don't have to, well, think much about. Though it is true that you are not consciously activating your muscles to lift your leg and place it the perfect distance in front of you, purposefully swinging your arms in opposition to your legs, or adjusting when you slip on a bit of loose gravel, the reality is that walking requires the precise coordination of hundreds of muscles, almost instantaneous evaluation of your environment, and constant adjustments to balance.

Consider all that goes on when you encounter a curb. First, you must accurately assess how far you are from the curb, how many steps it will take to get there and whether or not you need to shorten your stride. Next, you have to process the height of the curb to determine exactly how high you must lift your leg. Finally, as you scale Mount Curbside, you need to slow your pace and adjust your balance. All of this requires split-second analysis by your brain and directives to your muscles. For something that seems to be happening without conscious thought, there is a whole lot going on in that very busy brain of yours when you walk.

It might make you wonder, with all of this complicated analysis happening in real-time, how is it that you seem to think so clearly while you are walking? Recent research suggests it is due – at least in part – to your Default Mode Network.

Your Default Mode Network refers, generally, to your brain's auto-pilot system. Research suggests that, for some reason, switching on your Default Mode frees other parts of your brain to access memories, form connections, and gain deeper insight into your sense of self. Thus, when you walk, part of your brain is focused on putting one foot in front of the other, while the rest of your brain is free to roam, to think, and to problem solve, creating the perfect environment for thought.

As Ferris Jabr put it in a fantastic *New Yorker* article on the science of walking: "Because we don't have to devote much conscious effort to the act of walking, our attention is free to wander – to overlay the world before us with a parade of images from the mind's theater. This is precisely the kind of mental state that studies have linked to innovative ideas and strokes of insight."

Perhaps it is the Power of More Oxygen to our Brains

Walking increases the flow of oxygenated blood to the brain and provides the fuel it needs to function at its best. And brains need a lot of oxygen. In fact, though they comprise only about 2% of our body mass, our brains use about 20% of our oxygen consumption. And brains are highly sensitive to oxygen deprivation. So, the theory goes, the increased flow of oxygenated blood during a walk bathes the brain in the fuel it needs. By analogy, consider how your body feels when you haven't had enough to eat. Sluggish and with low energy. That is like your brain when you've been sitting too long. Lace up, take a walk, and nourish your brain with oxygenated blood flow.

Co-founder of Encore Retreats and former gymnast Lisa Waltuch found a way to take this theory to a whole 'nother level. "During graduate school," she explains, "when I got stuck on a problem, I would walk around my apartment on my hands. My thinking was ... getting more oxygen to my brain might help me come up with new ideas." She wasn't wrong, but for those of us who can't walk on our hands, a quick, brisk walk on our feet can do the trick.

Over time, your regular walking practice can also improve your overall cardiovascular health, continuing to improve the ability of your heart, lungs, and blood to deliver that all-important blood to your brain. Short-term and long-term improved oxygenation? Yes, please.

Perhaps it is the Boost in Brain-Derived Neurotrophic Factor (BDNF)

In considering the possible mechanisms by which walking helps our brain's function, growth, and plasticity, I'd be remiss not to mention BDNF, despite the fact that the research on the connection between BDNF and physical activity is nascent and somewhat inconclusive.

Brain-Derived Neurotrophic Factor, often referred to simply as BDNF, is a molecule related to many of the key brain functions we've been exploring, including memory and learning. First identified in the 1980s,

BDNF appears to be critical not just for our brains, but for our entire system in highly-complex ways that researchers continue working to understand. But one thing has become clear: BDNF is important and more of it is better.

If more BDNF is better, then the question becomes: how do we get more of it? Though the research on this is ongoing in both humans and animals, one way to increase our levels of BDNF may be physical activity.

In 2021, a team of researchers sought to analyze the existing research on the possible connection between physical activity and BDNF. They considered 907 different studies and ultimately included 49 in their evaluation. Noting inconsistencies in the characteristics of the many test subjects in those 49 studies, as well as variations in the type of the physical activities employed, they ultimately concluded that "studies performed in human populations appear to demonstrate a certain level of ambiguity" on the power of physical activity to stimulate BDNF while "in animal studies, the relationship between physical activity to regular exercise training does, indeed, in most cases, lead to an increase in BDNF concentration levels found in the blood."

And what about walking in particular? Has anyone considered walking specifically with regard to levels of BDNF? One small study looked at the power of walking on the BDNF levels of stroke survivors and concluded that 30 minutes of walking at a "moderate intensity" increased the participants' BDNF levels.

So does a regular walking practice help stimulate our bodies to produce BDNF? Perhaps.

Perhaps It Is the Power of Being in Nature

Attention Restoration Theory was first articulated by researchers Rachel and Stephen Kaplan in the late 1980s. They posited that being in nature can relieve mental fatigue and help to restore, among other things, your attention and decision-making capacity. The theory goes that certain behaviors deplete our stores of mental energy and diminish our concentration, but our focus and decision-making capacities can be replenished by spending time in nature.

Several decades of research has followed, which has confirmed that exposure to nature has a significant impact on your ability to focus, concentrate, and make good decisions.

To understand this more fully, I spoke with Cognitive Neuroscientist Dr. David Strayer who has sought to understand exactly what happens in the brain during these cognitive breaks. "When you take an unstructured walk in nature," he explained, "we see changes in the electrical systems in the brain. The parts of your brain that are involved in paying attention, orienting to stimuli and alerting to danger can become overworked. When people spend time walking in nature, we see these parts of the brain quiet, allowing them to rest and recover. This," he concluded, "appears to give you more cognitive capacity."

Conclusion

Despite the tremendous strides made over the past few decades in understanding how our brains work, they remain the most complex and mysterious facet of our physical bodies. Yet one thing has become clear: physical activity in general, and walking in particular, is very, very good for them.

Walking for Your Mood

**"Exercise is like taking an antidepressant;
not-exercising is like taking a depressant."**
Dr. Tal Ben-Shahar

I Was a Grumpy 16-Year-Old

It was one of those beautiful early spring days when the sky was blue, the sun was warm, and the world seemed full of possibilities. But not for me. I was 16 years old and I was grumpy. Really grumpy. Looking back, I have no idea why. It could have been a bad grade, a boy, or maybe the mean girls. I was 16, so it could have been nothing.

I crashed through the garage door, teenage angst written all over my face. My dad took one look at me and said, "Go for a walk, and then we'll talk."

A teacher, coach, and mentor to hundreds, my dad gets people. He has an incredible intuitive sense and he knows, perhaps better than anyone, the transformative power of physical activity. "Go for a walk," he repeated. "We'll talk when you get back."

I took his advice. I dropped my backpack on the red couch in the den and walked back out the door. Down our steep driveway, I took a right on West Shore Road, did a lap around Grenwolde Drive, then down Sinclair, and I finished up with the horseshoe that was Martin Court. A little over two miles.

I don't remember what was bugging me that day and I have no idea if my dad and I ever had a conversation about it. But I remember, with absolute clarity, the way my mood shifted between the moment I walked out the door and the moment I walked back in. I felt lighter, unburdened, energized and, well, happier.

That was the day I discovered that walking is a powerful antidote to a crappy day, though it would be several decades and thousands of miles before I learned about the research and the science behind what I discovered that day.

How is a walk such a powerful mood booster? What does the research teach us and what do the stories of thousands tell us?

The answer appears to involve several different mechanisms, and how those mechanisms affect each individual depends on each individual. As we will see, walking can fire up our positive hormones, tamp down our stress response, combat anxiety and depression, reduce rumination, reveal awe, boost energy, and improve sleep: All of which contribute to better outlooks, moods, and mental health.

The Power of Hormones

Hormones are not just the chemicals that cause teenagers to sprout body hair, pimples, and infuriating mood swings. Nor are they simply the chemicals that prompt desire. Rather, hormones include an extensive array of chemicals that are created by a host of our body's organs and drive a myriad of behaviors. Hormones are responsible for the stress response we will explore later in this chapter, impact how we process, use and store food, dictate how our bodies grow, and appear to be largely responsible for our addiction to slot machines and social media. And, yup, hormones drive much of our reproductive and sexual behavior.

Hormones can also help make us feel happy, connected, and calm.

Or not.

Which leads us to the connection between walking and hormones. As we will see momentarily, we have hormones and cannabinoids that promote positive feelings and are boosted by walking. Conversely, we have powerful hormones associated with stress and anxiety which can be reduced by walking.

Level Up the Positive Hormones

Thousands of years ago, philosopher Aristotle taught that the ultimate goal and purpose of life was to achieve happiness. More recently, the Dalai Lama reminded us that, "the purpose of our lives is to be happy."

Human beings have been chasing happiness for a long, long time.

Ask parents what they want for their children and most will answer, "I want them to be happy." Read any classic fairy tale and you'll be reminded that the goal is to reach the "happily ever after." Ask any therapist and they will tell you that most people arrive on their doorstep because they "just want to be happy."

We spend much of our lives chasing happiness, joy, and contentment. At least, we say we do. And yet over and over again, we do things that lead not to enduring joy and happiness, but momentary feel-good moments.

We self-medicate our sadness with donuts, social media, wine, or reality TV – all of which can be okay in small doses, but not so good in higher amounts. We invest our precious time pursuing *things* because of a misguided belief that more *things* will lead to more success, which will somehow deliver the happiness we believe lies on the other side of the next promotion or bigger bank account. And it is not entirely crazy. Higher status tickles the most ancient part of our brains, assuring us that it will make others like us more and make us more secure. Yet, over and over, research teaches that more money and more stuff does not lead to more happiness.

So what does? What exactly is happiness and how do we get it? In *Flourish*, Martin Seligman, who is often called the father of the positive psychology movement, notes that the problem with happiness is that it measures mood and cheerfulness, rather than overall well-being. The goal, he suggests, is not just to chase a good mood, but rather to embrace the elements of a meaningful, good life – minimize suffering *and* take positive steps to maximize flourishing.

Walking can help do that in many, many ways, starting with the benefits to the so-called "happiness hormones."

There are three primary hormones that contribute to feelings of happiness, satisfaction, and motivation – dopamine, serotonin and endorphins. They drive our productivity, which makes us feel good, which then encourages us to be more productive, which in turn keeps us moving forward in a uniquely human, positive cycle. They encourage us to connect with those we love, help regulate our mood, and dampen our pain response so that we can keep going. The better we understand these hormones, the better we can take steps to activate those that make us feel good. A robust body of research teaches that exercise, including walking, fires up all three of these hormones.

Dopamine

Dopamine is your chemical reward system. Sometimes referred to as our "feel-good neurotransmitter," it is released when we do things that satisfy us, from checking things off our to-do list, completing a project, getting a raise or a gold star, leveling up in a video game, eating that chocolate bar we crave, or seeing the "likes" grow on our social media posts. More recently, dopamine has been better understood as serving as a motivator that encourages us to keep moving toward things that we want, fueling our desire to learn new things, and one that encouraged our ancient ancestors to keep up the search for the elusive berry patch missed by the bears.

Serotonin

Serotonin does all sorts of things, and researchers continue to struggle to understand the precise mechanism by which it impacts our mental and emotional state. For our purposes, suffice to say that serotonin helps regulate our mood and contributes to positive feelings. It is the target of many antidepressants and appears to also impact our sleep cycle, making it even more critical to modulate our moods because sleep is essential to our physical, mental, and emotional well-being.

Endorphins

Endorphins reduce our perception of pain in a manner that is similar to how drugs like morphine work. Yup, that strong. Endorphins are the likely explanation for why sometimes an injury doesn't hurt until after a workout. Endorphins have also been credited with boosting moods, reducing stress, and even improving our immune response. Endorphins have long been credited with creating the so-called "runner's high" – that feeling of peace, calm, and downright euphoria that some people report following an extended bout of exercise. But scientists have begun to question this in large part because endorphins are molecules that don't cross the blood brain barrier. In other words, they don't appear to actually circulate into our brains.

Endocannabinoids

More recently, scientists have sought to unravel the mystery of endo-cannabinoids, which do cross the blood brain barrier and are believed to play a role in everything from sleep to bliss, and might actually be the chemicals that underlie the way exercise triggers positive feelings. Endocannabinoids are naturally occurring chemical compounds that are part of the endocannabinoid system, a complex system that researchers are just beginning to understand, but which has already been linked to a variety of physiological and cognitive processes including, pain, mood, appetite, sleep, chronic inflammation, and more.

You know what increases levels of endocannabinoids? Walking.

And ... a bonus hormone. As we will explore soon, walking with others boosts oxytocin, the hormone associated with connection, collaboration, and love.

Tamp Down the Stress Response

Imagine a time before human beings assigned numbers to the cycles of the seasons. The year is long. You are hungry. Your children are hungry, so you leave them in the cave and head out in search of food. It is a bright and sunny day and you start down a path you know well that leads to a lake where you have successfully fished in the past. Your stomach rumbles as you turn a corner and spot the lake in the distance. You've got this. But then you hear a different rumble in the bushes behind you. Bigger than a squirrel for sure, the hairs on the back of your neck stand on edge and, without conscious thought or decision, your body kicks into high gear. Your hypothalamus rings the alarm bell, triggering your adrenal glands to deliver a surge of adrenaline and cortisol. The adrenaline causes your heart rate to increase, your blood pressure to spike, and your strength to increase. The cortisol – often referred to as the body's "stress hormone" – dumps sugar into your bloodstream, fires up your brain, and diverts energy from systems you won't need while you battle the beast rustling in the bushes. You are not afraid because your fear response has been suppressed. There is no time for fear right now, only the decision of whether you should stay and fight, or turn and flee.

Your body's stress response has sharpened your senses, making you more responsive, agile, and stronger. You see better, hear better, and smell better. You are literally stronger. You are primed for battle.

But the beast in the bushes decides that you would not make for a tasty breakfast and turns the other direction. The battle never comes. Slowly, your breathing slows, your heart rate returns to normal, and you once again set your sights on the lake in front of you.

This stress response is a hard-wired survival mechanism. It is automatic: when you feel threatened, your body responds within seconds. And that is awesome. It shuts down systems unnecessary in battle, fires up those that are, and aligns everything we've got against a single threat. Your stress response is incredibly helpful when you are facing a life-threatening challenge.

But constant stress? We are not built for that.

Our stress response puts a serious strain on our bodies. It is there for a reason, but it is not there to be activated every day. Yet many of us are triggering our stress response far, far more often than nature intended. We feel our stress light up by things that don't cause an immediate threat to our existence, but by something mundane and every day: the guy who cut you off on the highway, a looming exam, a worry about a big work project. And then there are looming stressors that seem to be hanging over our heads: climate change, political upheaval, racial injustice, the threat of war, or another global pandemic. Millions of us are walking around in an almost constant state of humming stress alert, with heightened levels of cortisol coursing through our bodies a whole lot of the time.

That constant cortisol drip is not good for us. In fact, the evidence continues to mount that constant stress is really, really bad for us. Heightened levels of cortisol have been linked to:

- Anxiety;
- Depression;
- Stomach and digestive problems;
- Weight gain;
- Worry;
- Irritability; and
- Insomnia.

Guess what? Walking just 20 minutes – especially outdoors in nature – significantly reduces cortisol levels and tamps down your stress response.

Our stress response is one of our most potent biological systems. It is complicated and it is valuable. The goal is not to live without any stress. That would be impossible and would create lives that were neither as challenging nor as fun as most of us would choose. Rather, the goal is to teach our bodies to know when that stress response is needed and teach it to lay dormant when it is not.

Walking can help do that.

Walking Helps Combat Depression and Fight Anxiety

We often talk about depression and anxiety in a single breath, as if they are the same thing. Both are considered "mood disorders" and, for sure, both can impact the quality of our lives. And for some people, and at some times, depression and anxiety can coexist with one amplifying the other. But they are not the same thing.

Depression

When my son was about 14, he retreated into his room, his computer, and his video games. Months went by. He was growing like a weed and within a year, he was a full head taller than his peers; a situation that corrected itself by 11th grade. He was angry and sad. His energy and his humor were gone and his light had dimmed.

He describes his journey through depression in this way:

Imagine you're a fisherman. Not a commercial fisherman, but an avid hobbyist. You spend most weekends knee-deep in a lake, river, stream, or any body of water you can find. You love catching fish. You bring a tacklebox with every kind of bait, lure, bob, and line imaginable. After every trip you tell your friends about your best catch, how the weather was, and your next plans to go fishing. Your friends and family are sup-portive and sometimes they even join you.

Then one trip you don't catch any fish. Not a single one. You think, "Hmm, that's odd. I've done everything right. I'm at the same spot I always am, using my best line and lures, where are the fish?" Maybe you mention to your friends that you didn't catch anything. They say, "Ah well, bad luck, I guess." But it's not sitting right with you. There's always fish. Maybe it was just a fluke.

The next weekend comes and you try a different lake. You change the lure too. Still no fish. You even stay longer. The sun has set, the birds have grown quiet, and you're still standing there, rod in hand, fishless. You tell your friends and they are surprised. 'How could you not catch any fish? Did you use the right lure? Have you tried the river? What about live bait?' On and on they ask questions and give suggestions that you already know should enable you to catch fish. But still you don't. No matter what you try, you never catch another fish.

What do you do? This is your favorite hobby. Or, was your favorite hobby. Would you continue trying? Put on the waders, the sunscreen, reorganize your tacklebox and your lines, just go to a lake or a river that you know once provided bounties of fish just to stand there?

My son loved reading, playing video games, hanging out with friends, all the usual teenager stuff. Until one day, he didn't.

"When you're depressed," he explains, "doing the things you enjoyed in the past gives you no joy. Since nothing feels worth doing, you decide to do nothing. And that feels very reasonable."

I read everything I could on depression and teens. I orchestrated my days to minimize the amount of time he was home alone. I roasted walnuts and grilled salmon and loaded our refrigerator with foods that have been shown to help support mood and mental health.

We pushed, gently, towards therapy which he resisted until one day, frustrated with his own misery, he agreed. Sure, we could have forced him – and we were close – but I knew my kid. He is stubborn and strong and can be contrary, and I feared that if he wasn't onboard, no amount of therapy would help.

Off we went to our initial family session with Bettina. "What I'm trying to figure out," I said, "is this normal teenage angst or something more? Just how worried should we be?"

Over the following months, we all sought to answer that question. Finally Bettina suggested we consult with a doctor. "I think there is more here than typical teenage moodiness," she said. "I have someone I would recommend."

After several sessions, the psychiatrist called us all into his office. "There's a continuum," he explained. "And I believe that your son is tipped over the midpoint from teenage malaise into depression. I think it is worth trying medication and seeing if it helps." We looked at our son.

"It's up to you," I said. "You shouldn't have to feel this way. You deserve to feel happy. Heck, you deserve to feel. I say we try it. But again, it's up to you." I knew that we needed his buy-in for any treatment to be successful.

"Okay," he said after a long pause. "Let's try it."

The doctor did a DNA scrape of his cheek to help inform the choice of medication. "There's no guarantee that we will get it right the first time," he cautioned.

But we did. He started with the lowest possible dose and within ten days, the light had returned to my son's eyes.

Depression is a scary beast that sits at the intersection of mental, physical, and emotional well-being. It has no easy answers. Medication helps some, but not others, and a thousand factors play into its management. Every person who wrestles with depression is unique and there is no quick fix.

If you have any of the warning signs for depression – if you feel sad more often than not, have lost interest in the things that typically bring you joy, if you feel helpless, worthless or hopeless, if your sleep has changed (sleeping much more, or much less), if you think about harming yourself, cry frequently, feel depleted, if most days feel like a long, unhappy slog, or if that little voice inside you is telling you you shouldn't feel this way or that something isn't right, run – don't walk – towards professional help. And if the first person with whom you consult doesn't help, try another. Because there are people who can. *

Walking is not a panacea or a quick fix. But study after study, and story after story, have shown that walking can be a powerful tool to help combat depression both by ameliorating current symptoms and helping to protect against future depressive episodes.

In one such study, a team of researchers set out to determine whether physical activity can be used as therapeutic means for acute and chronic depression. The researchers noted that while medical treatment can be effective at treating depression, they estimated that only 10 to 25% of those affected receive treatment, either due to lack of resources, lack of access to providers, or lingering social stigma associated with mental health. They reviewed and synthesized dozens of studies, papers, and articles in an effort to understand the interplay

* If you believe you might be suffering from depression, there is help available. If you are uncertain where to start, the US Department of Health and Human Services has a free, confidential help line that can provide you with information and connect you with local treatment facilities, support groups, and community organizations. They can be reached 24/7 at 800-662-4357 (HELP). The National Suicide Prevention Hotline is 800-273-8255.

between exercise and mental health. They concluded that "exercise and physical activity have beneficial effects on depression symptoms that are comparable to those of antidepressant treatments."

What about walking in particular? In 2022, researchers synthesized 15 different studies which included more than 190,000 individuals and concluded that, "activity equivalent to 2.5 hours of brisk walking per week was associated with 25% lower risk of depression, and at half that dose, the risk was 18% lower compared with no activity."

None of this would come as a surprise to Sharon Carter* for whom walking has always been a salve. "When I was in high school, I began my journey with anxiety and depression. People didn't really understand and there wasn't as much focus on mental health in the '90s. We lived by a small lake, and often, at midnight, under that anonymity of darkness, I would go for a walk. It was my escape and I'm not sure if I loved it or if it loved me, but I know it helped."

Decades later, Sharon would return to her walking practice following the most difficult time of her life. "My eldest child began struggling with major depression. She was a cheerleader and began having a hard time with her friends and her coach. She had started cutting, but I thought it was under control and she saw a therapist, so it was all good, right? Wrong. There were tears and a breakdown and an admission of suicidal thoughts. We went to the ER and waited 12 hours to get a bed in a mental health facility. I signed papers and left my child. This was the beginning of my spiral.

"For the next three years, I became a shell. I was determined to make my child want to live. I was determined to fix my baby with so much love. I dragged her to therapy, fought doctors for medication changes, and argued diagnoses. I invaded her private spaces, read her journals, analyzed her artwork, and took away anything that could possibly be broken and made sharp. This was my mission, my raison d'être. I was miserable and I made my child miserable right along with me.

"Brooke came to me when she was 16 and told me that she was transgender, and had changed his name to Brian. I wasn't ready for that and didn't trust it. I thought it was just another ploy for attention. We began to fight and one day, he packed his boxes and left my home to go live with his mostly absent father. I was crushed. I cried for months. I wallowed in self-pity.

"For three years, I had been under so much stress, both real and self-imposed, that my joints ached, my skin was pale, I was constantly sick, my hair was falling out, and I had gained 70 pounds. I needed to do something

* Both the mom and child's names have been changed to protect their anonymity.

other than cry. I needed to do something good for myself. I wasn't getting anywhere on the path I was on. And so, like I had done as a teenager, I started walking. I used my miles to cry and reflect and think. I craved the peace and serenity this walking practice gave me. It saved my sanity, helped me rediscover my worth, and allowed me to become a better mother. One year later, we are continuing to repair our relationship. I have become closer to my child. I have been more successful at my job. I have learned grace and dignity."

Sharon is hardly alone. Kelly Sue Warden has also learned to leave her stress on a walking trail. "I've been on antidepressants and migraine medication for years. A lot of medicine has side effects. I told my doctor that I wanted to be off of the meds. I read that exercise could help with depression. I started walking and heard someone suggest walking with the intention of leaving your stress on the trail. That's what I do. On every walk, I think about all the stress in my life and then I leave it all there.

"Because of my walking practice, my doctor has weaned me off of antidepressants. I'm happier and healthier than I have been in years. I have more energy, which I need with two grown kids, a granddaughter, and an insulin-dependent diabetic husband to care for. It's been 22 years of putting myself last. I still do everything I can for them, but I carve out time for myself. Walking has saved my life."

Anxiety

Let's start with the reality that everyone experiences anxiety from time to time. When you are late for an appointment and you feel your heart rate climbing as you fight the temptation to tailgate the little blue Honda doing just under the speed limit. The tight, uncomfortable feeling when you walk into a party where you don't know a soul. The dread as you sit in a doctor's waiting room awaiting the results of last week's biopsy.

Anxiety is normal. Except when it is not. Except when your system overreacts to typical anxiety-provoking situations. Or when an overactive imagination creates anxiety producing situations out of the day-to-day flotsam and jetsam of life. Or any of the dozen different causes and symptoms of an anxiety disorder.

My anxiety can fire up as a result of a thousand different things: being late, contemplating my own mortality, worrying about my family's physical safety, confronting months when money in doesn't keep up with money out, or that blasted blue Honda keeping me from getting where I need to go. My breathing becomes shallow, my thoughts race, and that weird tingly feeling runs down my arms. If I pay attention, I can feel the adrenaline and cortisol coursing through my body.

Everyone experiences anxiety at times, but for more than 40 million adults, those anxiety levels cross the line into anxiety disorders, which are the most common psychiatric illnesses in the U.S.

Walking helps. A lot.

In fact, from studies cited by the Anxiety and Depression Association of America,"regular exercise works as well as medication for some people to reduce symptoms of anxiety and depression, and the effects can be long lasting. One vigorous exercise session can help alleviate symptoms for hours, and a regular schedule may significantly reduce them over time."

How?

Researchers believe the anxiety-ameliorating effect of exercise is likely a combination of things: the boost in happiness hormones, the reduction in stress hormones, positive impacts on brain health, improvements in self-esteem, reduction in rumination, benefits of being in nature, improvement in sleep, and boost to your immune system – all of which we will explore in chapters to come.

In short, while they aren't 100% sure how physical activity and walking helps to combat depression and anxiety, researchers are quite confident that it does.

A final, important reminder

An anxiety and depression disorder requires professional help. If anxiety or depression are interfering with your ability to function or enjoy life, prompting thoughts of hopelessness or suicide, causing you to turn to drugs or alcohol, I implore you to get the professional help you need to live the life you deserve. *

Rumination and Walking

Search the verb "ruminate" in the dictionary and you will find familiar definitions. To ruminate means to think deeply about something. To contemplate, or examine it repeatedly in your mind. To ponder. Search the noun "rumination" and the first definitions you find include deeply considered thoughts or ideas. This all sounds good, doesn't it? Especially in our fast-moving world, the idea of taking the time to deeply contemplate thoughts, ideas, and questions can be a luxury. We romanticize the great thinkers of history and picture them considering the world's most important questions in profound and thoughtful ways. We imagine Ralph Waldo Emerson and Henry David Thoreau drifting on clouds of contemplation, seeking understanding.

Rumination seems like a good thing. And it is, until it's not.

You know those nights when the dog (or partner) wakes you up with their snoring at 2:00 a.m., you nudge them awake and roll them over, fluff your pillow and try to get back to sleep, but then you start thinking about the stupid thing you said to your boss during your morning meeting, the moment when you snapped at your daughter after school, how stupid you were not to have taken the *other* job when you graduated from college, or maybe that one time you inadvertently insulted the most popular girl in school when you were 16? "*I'm an idiot,*" you think, as these negative thoughts swirl repeatedly in circles around your mind. 'Round and 'round and no matter how hard you try, you can't let them go.

You are ruminating. And not in a good way.

In psychology, rumination – referred to as "depressive rumination" "brooding" or "morbid rumination" – is what happens when we repeatedly replay a problem or a negative thought over and over again. Typically, those negative thoughts relate to feelings of inadequacy, failure, or low self worth.

Rumination is closely aligned with depression and anxiety. It has been called a "silent mental health problem" and too much brooding and ruminating has been shown to be part and parcel of the dark spiral that is depression and anxiety. Brain scans have shown that rumination lights up activity in your prefrontal cortex, a part of your brain that is involved in how emotions are regulated.

How do you stop ruminating? Like all of the answers relating to mental health, there is no easy, one-size fits all answer. Rumination can be difficult to disrupt and can be an indicator of more serious mental health issues. But most of us find ourselves ruminating on the negative from time to time, and on those days taking your brain for a walk can help. Bonus points for walking in nature.

Walking Can Help You Process Difficult Things

Grief is a complicated thing. While everyone experiences grief at some point in their lives, how they process and move through that experience is as unique as they are. People in the throes of grief may experience impaired concentration, insomnia, aggression, depression, or post-traumatic stress and, while researchers have identified "a multitude of factors which can influence how a person grieves," everyone's grief journey is different. For many, like Paige Hess, walking offers a useful tool to help move through their grief.

"My walking journey began in 2011, months after losing my mom to cancer," Paige explains. "My sisters and I signed up for a Susan G. Komen 3-day 60-mile walk. We chose the last walk of the year, giving us ten months to train. I walked through my grief, spending many Saturdays walking down a country road in tears remembering my mom and thinking about how proud she would be of all of us doing this in her honor. Ten months later, my sisters and I flew to Dallas. I walked 57 of the 60 miles – hitching a ride for the last three. The walk was very therapeutic, emotionally and physically.

"Walking is more than putting one foot in front of the other. Walking is spending time with my thoughts and decompressing the day. It is 'me' time. It is proving to myself that I am so much more and that the best is yet to come. Walking is fuel for the soul," she said.

For others, like Martha, walking offered the privacy she needed while grieving the loss of her mother. "With two little kids always underfoot," she explains, "my solo walks gave me the time to think and to feel that I didn't have while I was home. My kids knew I was grieving and they were grieving too. I didn't want to hide my grief from them, but I didn't want to completely fall apart in front of them either."

How? Why? So many reasons.

Walking gives you the time and space to process emotions while powering up your brain to function at its best and firing up your positive hormones. Perhaps those happiness hormones provide a buffer that enables you to let yourself feel what you need to feel. Maybe walking in nature gives you a chance to see your grief through the lens of the vastness of the world. Perhaps it is something else entirely. But however it works, Paige and Martha are only two of the many, many people who have walked through their grief.

Walking Helps You Discover Awe

We didn't travel much when I was a kid. My dad coached sports and taught middle school; my mom was a part-time dance teacher. While we had everything we needed, there wasn't much left for travel and my parents weren't the camping types. So, other than a couple of weekends in Atlantic City and one memorable family trip to Miami, I don't recall any other childhood trips. It wasn't until my late 20s that I ventured to the western United States.

It was the first week of April and my then-boyfriend and I headed to Park City, Utah, for a week of spring skiing. It was beautiful, but skiing through the spring slush was exhausting. By day three we had an idea: let's drive down to Arches National Park and go hiking. A four-hour drive landed me at the mouth of the first national park I'd ever visited. Everything, from the deep orange-red color of the rocks to the soaring sandstone arches, was awe-inspiring.

Awe. Inspiring.

The feeling I experienced at Arches National Park was a full decade before psychologists began to explore the emotion they have dubbed "awe." Awe has been described as "an overwhelming, self-transcendent sense of wonder and reverence in which you feel a part of something that is vast, larger than you, and that transcends your understanding of the world." Awe can be found in those moments when we become captivated by the enormity, the beauty, and seeming impossibility of "it all."

Researchers are just beginning to understand the impact that awe has on us.

Awe makes us feel small in the grand scheme of the universe, while at the same time, helps us feel connected to something larger than ourselves. This paradox is a cornerstone of awe. Experiencing awe results in lower stress, reduced inflammation, and increased joy. We tend to be more curious, more open to new ideas, and more deeply engaged with others. Awe can also decrease our attachment to material things, expand our perception of time, and make life feel more satisfying.

More joy. Less stuff. Improved health. The sense that we have more time. Sounds great, but how do we get more awe? Do we need to travel to exotic, unfamiliar, epic places? Must we hike to Mount Everest base camp, windsurf in Maui, parachute into a volcano, or sail around Alaskan glaciers? Not necessarily. Turns out, we can simply walk for awe.

In 2020, Professor Virginia Strum led a team of researchers from the University of California to explore the impact of what they coined "Awe Walks" on the emotional state of older adults.

The researchers recruited 60 healthy adults between the ages of 60 and 90 and assigned them to either an "awe walk" group or a "control walk" group. Both groups were instructed to take weekly 15-minute walks outdoors for eight weeks with one key difference: the "awe walk" group was encouraged to vary the locations of their walks when possible and was given some direction on how to tap into their "sense of wonder" while they walked. "We kept it simple. We explained what awe is and asked them to shift their focus during their walks to look outwards and be curious," Professor Sturm explains. The "control walk" group was given no additional instruction.

Participants completed written surveys about their walks and how they felt, as well as other daily surveys designed to provide insight into whether or not their walks impacted their emotional state, even when they were not actively walking. They were also asked to take selfies, which the researchers used to evaluate their "smile intensity" and "self-size." Here's what they found.

Those who had been instructed to look for awe on their walks experienced "significantly higher awe" than those who had not been given such instruction. They reported greater feelings that they were part of something larger than themselves, and higher levels of positive emotions like compassion and joy. The awe group smiled bigger and the more walks they took, the bigger those smiles became. "We coded the facial expressions from more than a thousand selfies using an objective system," Professor Sturm explains. "Over time, the smiles of the awe group became bigger."

Professor Sturm told me that even she was surprised at how well it worked. "We discovered that it's not that hard to get people to experience awe on their walks and that the benefits of awe walks accumulate over time. Awe helps us to feel connected to others and to the world and encourages prosocial behavior including gratitude, compassion, and kindness. In short, it helps us be better humans."

Lexi Hidalgo is a 22-year-old podcaster and social media personality whose frank, authentic, and honest voice resonates deeply with her more than three million followers and fans – most of whom are teenage girls seeking context for their feelings and advice navigating their always on, social-media soaked culture. Reminding millions of girls that it is okay to be themselves and that life can be both hard and beautiful is work that Lexi loves, but it is also work that can, if she's not careful, take a toll. "It can be draining," Lexi admits, "and I've burned out a few times."

Over the years, Lexi has discovered tools that help. Among them? Walking, the power of which she discovered inadvertently and with a fair bit of skepticism.

"There were three of us living together in Hawaii. It was a very difficult time for me, I was wrestling with depression and anxiety and had some hard things to work out," Lexi explains. "One of my friends would go for walks all the time. And I was like, *'Why is she doing this?'*"

Nevertheless, Lexi began walking around her neighborhood or down by the beach. "These walks gave me time to be alone with myself and I discovered that was when I found the most valuable thoughts, the most valuable ideas, and the most peace of mind. I would walk whenever I was super anxious just because it made me feel better." Sometimes, she'd call people and catch up with friends, but other times, this always-on millennial would walk without her phone, a practice that Lexi believes has had a huge impact on her mental health.

"I would simply look around and be present wherever I was. If I was on the beach, I would pay attention to the way different waves crashed or the way the clouds moved. If I was walking around my neighborhood, I would focus on the different dogs that walked by, or a mother and daughter unloading groceries from the car, or a father and son playing football in the front yard. I'd notice the tiny little things that I didn't typically pay attention to. It taught me an appreciation for nature and for life and gave me an understanding that everything else continues to go on in the world, even if I sit still. I don't know why that made me feel good, but it did. It made me feel content."

Without putting a label on it, without going out to actively look for it, Lexi discovered the power of an intentional walk to deliver a healthy dose of awe.

Better Than A Shot of Espresso

You know those days when you've done nothing but sit in front of your computer cranking out PowerPoint slides, spreadsheets, or stories? Or those days when you have been barraged by a constant stream of "Mom, Mom, Mom, Mom?" Whatever the cause, those days when 4:00 p.m. rolls around and you realize you are completely and utterly exhausted and yet you have barely moved?

"Ah," you think, "what I need is a cup of coffee to perk me up." Or a chocolate chip cookie. Or maybe two chocolate chip cookies.

While a hit of caffeine could help, research has consistently shown that a walk is likely to help more in both the short and long-term.

It's physics. Well, sort of.

Sir Isaac Newton, one of history's most brilliant mathematicians and physicists stated in his first law of motion that a body at rest will remain at rest unless acted upon by an outside force, and that a body in motion will remain in motion unless acted upon by an outside force. Now, he was talking about physical objects, like a rock rolling down a hill, not about human bodies. But the analogy applies: if you are at rest and are not moving, there is much that is acting upon you to keep you at rest. Your circulation is low, your happy hormones are low, your metabolism is low, and your energy is not flowing. When you get moving, your system springs into action. Your circulation fires up, bringing blood flow, oxygen, and glucose to your muscles and organs – including your brain. The net result is ... more energy.

In fact, a study conducted by researchers at the University of Georgia in Athens compared the impact of a low intensity, 10-minute walk in a stairwell to the impact of the consumption of 50 mg of caffeine – just slightly less than is in a typical shot of espresso. Those who took the walk felt more energized than those who consumed the caffeine. This study doesn't stand alone in the research field – many others have confirmed the energy boosting effect of movement.

Walking doesn't just help you defeat the late afternoon energy doldrums for the short-term. A regular walking practice can have a profound impact on your long-term energy levels for many of the reasons we've discussed thus far. Among them? Walking helps combat depression. And it is no surprise to hear that depression itself is an energy sapper. And as we will discover, walking helps improve your cardiovascular system, maintain a healthy weight, and get better sleep at night. All of which are closely aligned with your energy levels.

And Then There Are Just Those Days

I was having a day. One of those days when every little thing seemed to go wrong and every person I encountered presented a problem, a challenge, or an annoyance. The overpriced coffee was cold and the barista surly. A Range Rover stole my parking spot and not ten minutes later, another one cut me off. I found myself hanging up on the customer service rep who clearly needed some education in customer service.

But then I realized if every single person I encountered during the course of my day was annoying me in some way, chances are, it wasn't them, it was me. Somehow, I was pouring out negativity, attracting negativity, or viewing everything through a lens of negativity. I needed an energy adjustment. I needed to derail my day to get it back on track.

I canceled an afternoon call (which I'm sure was for the best because heaven knows what would have happened had I tried to lead a team meeting), grabbed my favorite sneakers, and hit the woods for three, quiet miles.

Energy, mood, and mindset all adjusted.

A walk is a powerful antidote to a crappy day.

Walking for Your Body

"Walking is man's best medicine."
Hippocrates

I Was Right ... And I Was Wrong

The year was 1990 and I was a first-year associate at a huge law firm. As a commercial litigator, I represented big companies in big lawsuits. I spent long hours in the law library, argued motions in court, locked myself in conference rooms to write complex legal briefs, long-hand, on yellow legal pads, and carried the bags of the senior partner to argue one of those briefs before the Federal Court of Appeals. I remember he took a limo to the courthouse. I took a cab. This was long, long before Uber. My work was simultaneously heady and challenging and mind-numbing and dull.

One day, all of the first year associates were instructed to attend a full-day accounting seminar. The thinking, I assume, was that our job often required us to understand our clients' financial records and to decipher those of our adversaries. So on a beautiful June Saturday, we piled into a large conference room on the eleventh floor of a big-six accounting firm. There were windows overlooking Third Avenue. I think the windows were their mistake.

The two accountants leading the seminar kicked it off at 9:00 on the button – they were accountants afterall. For the next three hours, they droned on about balance sheets, debits, credits, and I have no idea what else. Finally, noon came and we were released for a one-hour lunch break.

I walked out of the building into the spring sunshine and bought a sandwich from the deli across the street, which I ate in a small park watching a few kids play on the swings. With 20 minutes left, I wandered into a Gap store, bought a perfect white t-shirt and then returned to the conference room for four more hours of accounting. I flopped down in a chair next to my friend Marissa, opened my notebook, and looked up.

The two men began the afternoon lecture. Above their heads was a big, round clock. It was one of those older clocks with a second-hand that moved with little jerky movements – click, click, click. I watched 15 seconds click by and realized, with a sudden jolt of clarity, that my life was now 15 seconds shorter. I had no idea – and still have no idea – exactly how much time I have to be with the people I love, make an impact on the world, and do the things that make my heart sing, but I knew that my time here is fixed and that I had 15 seconds less of it.

I closed my notebook and grabbed the blue Gap bag from the floor. "Where are you going?" Marissa hissed.

"I'm leaving," I said. And I slipped out of that conference room, rode the elevator to the lobby, stepped into the sunshine and walked home.

My compulsion to leave that conference room was based on a belief that the number of seconds we have on this earth are fixed and finite. I was both right and wrong.

Yes, we have only a certain number of years, days, hours, and seconds to do all that we long to do. But it turns out that we can do things that can dramatically impact how many of those years, weeks, days, hours, minutes, and seconds we get. Of course, there are no guarantees. Illness and accidents happen every day even when we "do everything right."

But the research proves, time and again, that we have countless opportunities to make choices and take actions that can add not just years, but quality years, to our lives.

And one of the most powerful things we can do?

Walk.

Over the past several decades, research has proven that exercise can add years to our lives and that one of the best lifetime forms of exercise is walking. Walking has been shown to materially reduce our risk of high-blood pressure, high-cholesterol, heart disease, obesity, and diabetes. It can strengthen our bones, combat osteoporosis, and reduce our risk of several types of cancers. Walking supports our immune system and helps regulate healthy sugar levels. As we discussed in the chapter on brain heath, walking reduces our risk of dementia and Alzheimer's and helps keep us active, mobile, and engaged with the world around us, which are key markers for a long and happy life.

As my 92-year-old dad said, "As I've gotten older, I've become even more convinced that exercise is the key to my longevity." Yup Dad, as usual, you are spot on.

Let's dig in.

Yes, Walking Counts

"Walking doesn't count as exercise," a woman named Elizabeth said. "I mean, it's just walking."

I had just completed a live interview about the magic of walking and we opened the floor for conversation, beginning with the audience's thoughts and impressions about exercise in general and walking in particular. That's when Elizabeth piped up. "Exercise is, well, *exercise*," she repeated. "And walking is just, well, walking."

Just walking. Just lifting one foot, extending it in front of you while you momentarily balance on a single leg. While your heart pumps blood to those working legs, your arms swing in perfect cadence in opposition to your footfalls, your brain processes thousands of pieces of data to trigger micro-adjustments to hundreds of muscles. Over and over and over again, an average of 2,000 times for each mile you walk.

It's just walking. But it's also not.

Consider the muscles that work while you walk. Think it is just your legs? Think again.

Sure, your legs are pressed into service with every step: your quads, glutes, hamstrings, and calves, along with all of those tiny stabilizer muscles you've never heard of. In fact, virtually every muscle in your lower body is activated while you walk and when you walk barefoot, you add the two dozen muscles associated with your feet.

There's more. To walk, you must remain upright, stable, and balanced, activating your pelvis, core, and back. And remember that arm swing? Add in arms and shoulders, especially when you "power walk" or take a pair of walking poles along.

And last, but certainly not least – perhaps the most important muscle of all, the one without which there is no more walking, no more loving, no more anything – your heart.

All of those muscles, working in perfect coordination.

Does walking count as exercise? Absolutely. Yet, we have been sold a bill of goods by what I affectionately call the "fitness industrial complex." Media, advertisers, and tens of thousands of fitness companies have told us, in subtle and not so subtle ways, that "exercise" and "fitness" look a certain way.

Scroll social media or turn on your television and you quickly become convinced that fitness is thin women in close-fitting yoga pants and crop tops, their hair in high ponytails, precariously balanced in crow pose, twisted into eagle pose, pounding the pavement, or bopping to the rhythm. And the men? There you'll discover shaved chests and bulging biceps, 200 pounds of metal hoisted over their heads, or panting through a triathlon. Though we are finally beginning to see women picking up and putting down heavy things (resistance training is fantastic for both women and men), the message remains clear: one must master heavy weights, run marathons, feel the burn, and push the limits. No pain, no gain.

It is no wonder that millions of Americans have decided that "fitness is not for me," hundreds have told me they "hate exercise," and so many have concluded, "Why bother?"

"I've joined three gyms in my life," another woman shared during that interview. "And never stepped foot into any one of them. I'm just not the gym-going type and I always thought that meant there was no way for me to 'get exercise.' Hearing that walking counts? Well, that changes everything."

Yes, walking counts. That doesn't mean that other activities don't count as well. Ideally, we all stretch and maintain our mobility. We all engage in some kind of resistance training. We all play and explore. Perhaps we swim or dance or bike or CrossFit or play pickleball. But the fact that other things are also good for us doesn't mean that walking isn't.

There's research to prove it. Lots and lots of research.

In 2017, a team of researchers sought to compare the reduction in mortality from walking versus other types of physical activity. They focused on walking because it is "free, does not require special training, and can be done almost anywhere." Thus, "better understanding the mortality benefit associated with walking has important implications for tailoring public health messages, increasing population-wide levels of walking and decreasing health costs, especially among older adults."

They analyzed the relationship between walking – in the absence of other types of physical activity – and mortality among 140,000 adults between the ages of 47 and 89 and found that walking between four hours and six hours per week was associated with a 20% lower mortality risk. And the news kept getting better: walking six or more hours per week "was associated with a 29% lower all-cause death rate compared with being insufficiently active."

29% reduced risk of death.

A similar result was reached in another large study that spanned nearly six years and included 73,743 women between the ages of 50 and 79.

The researchers noted that while physical activity has been associated with a reduced risk of cardiovascular disease, data for women and members of minority groups have been limited. "Moreover, the specific role of walking, the most common form of exercise among women, has been addressed only minimally." The researchers set out to change this by comparing the impact of walking with that of vigorous exercise in the prevention of cardiovascular disease.

They noted that *both* "walking and vigorous exercise are associated with substantial reductions in the incidence of cardiovascular events," and concluded that "women who either walked briskly or exercised vigorously at least 2.5 hours per week had a risk reduction of approximately 30 percent."

Walking only.

So yes, Elizabeth, walking counts.

Why is it important to recognize that walking "counts" as exercise? Because what we think about how we move impacts how our bodies respond to that movement.

In a famous study, Harvard Professors Dr. Alia Crum and Dr. Ellen Langer tested what, if anything, happens to us physically when we realize that things we do "count as exercise." The protocol was simple and the results profound.

84 hotel housekeepers were separated into two groups: the "informed group" and the "control group." Members of the informed group were told that the work they did was exercise sufficient to satisfy the Surgeon General's recommendations for an active, healthy lifestyle. It was explained that exercise does not need to be hard or painful to be good for their health and they were given specifics about how their work cleaning hotel rooms – from vacuuming to cleaning bathrooms – was, in fact, exercise.

The control group was not provided with any such instruction or education.

Both group's workload remained constant during the 30 days prior to and during the 30 days of the study. For the informed group, the only thing that changed was their understanding that the work they did "counted" as exercise. This single mindful shift resulted in "remarkable improvement" in several physiological measures. After only 4 weeks, the group that had been told that they were exercising while working lost an average of 2 pounds, 6 lowered their blood pressure, and 7 saw improvements in body-fat percentage, BMI, and hip-to-waist ratio. These were meaningful changes, especially considering that they occurred in just 4 weeks.

Knowing that walking "counts" as exercise matters.

Biological vs. Chronological Age and Telo-Whats?

Before recorded time, I don't know if human beings counted their chronological age. Did they make a notch on the wall of their cave for each winter they survived? Maybe, but probably not. The notion of keeping track of our years on this earth seems to be something we likely developed when we started formally counting those years. Since then, we've been a little bit obsessed with chronological age. How old was the Egyptian Boy-King Tutankhamun when he reigned? What was the average life-span before the industrial revolution? How 'bout after? Why do people in the Mediterranean tend to live longer and what about the seemingly magic Blue Zones – regions of the planet where more people have the chance to celebrate their 100th birthday than in other places? We count the years and memorialize them with cards and candles.

Over the past few years, scientists have begun asking a more nuanced question: what is your *biological* age? Though closely associated with your chronological age (measured strictly as the number of years you've been alive) your biological age is different. If your chronological age is, say, 50, what about the quality of your blood, bones, brain, and DNA? Do they exhibit the markers of a typical 50-year-old, or are they more akin to those of a 65-year-old or, better yet, a 35-year-old?

One of the markers of biological age is your telomeres.

Telomeres are sections of your DNA that sit at the end of your chromosomes. They hold critical information that helps cells divide and replicate. As we age, our telomeres become shorter, and the shorter they become, the more difficult it is for them to do their job and for our cells to regenerate. Hence, the longer your telomeres, the younger your "biological age."

That is a tremendous simplification of a very complex scheme, but the bottom line is this: the length of our telomeres is a key marker of our health and longevity.

While many, many factors impact telomere length, recent studies have identified a relationship between physical activity in general, and walking in particular, on telomere length.

In 2020, Dr. Larry A. Tucker of Brigham Young University investigated a possible connection between walking and telomere length. He and his team analyzed data of more than 5,800 adults and discovered that those who walked at least 150 minutes per week had "significantly longer telomeres than those who did no regular walking," and that individuals who walked for more than the 150 minutes had telomeres longer than those who walked less than the 150 minutes per week standard. In drawing this conclusion, Dr. Tucker adjusted for many other variables, including the participants' participation in other forms of activity. He concluded that, "in short, it appears that regular walking explains differences in telomere length better than other forms of activity considered collectively."

And the news keeps getting better. A 2022 study of more than 400,000 adults confirmed a causal link between walking pace and telomere length, revealing that a "faster walking pace is indeed likely to lead to a younger biological age as measured by telomeres."

At the time of this writing, this research is in its infancy, as research-ers have yet to identify the mechanism by which more walking is related to telomere length. Is it causative, or merely correlative? Perhaps people with lower biological ages simply walk more. But with all of the extensive benefits of walking for your mind, mood, and body, I am confident that there is more to it than coincidence.

Heart Health

Ask people which disease they fear and most will answer "cancer." Breast cancer. Blood cancer. Lung cancer. The cancer whispered in that dark, knowing tone: pancreatic cancer.

Don't get me wrong – cancer is terrifying and we will explore walking and the reduction in cancer risk shortly – but by the numbers, heart disease kills far more people than all types of cancers combined. According to the CDC, heart disease accounts for one in every five deaths, taking the lives of about 697,000 people each year in the US alone. It is the leading cause of death for both men and women.

So, if we want to stay alive, and stay healthy, it pays to look first at ways to keep our hearts healthy. One of the best? Walking.

Bus Drivers versus Bus Conductors

Somewhere around 400 BC, Hippocrates, long-considered the father of Western medicine, declared that "walking is man's best medicine." But it wasn't until the 1950s that doctors and researchers began to collect data suggesting he was right. It started with London's iconic double-decker buses.

One of the first, and oft-cited, studies to demonstrate the impact of regular physical activity on heart disease, health, and longevity was conducted in London in the early 1950s. Researchers sought to "un-cover social factors" that might be contributing to a notable rise in heart disease. To do so, they evaluated the incidence of heart disease between two groups of approximately 31,000 men between the ages of 35 and 64 who were employed by London's transportation system.

Group one included the bus drivers, whose work was largely sedentary. Group two included the bus conductors, whose work involved walking around the bus collecting tickets, including climbing the stairs to the buses' upper level. In most other respects, the two groups were similar, sharing similar socio-economic status, work hours, and ages.

The researchers considered the incidence of heart-disease as well as the outcomes: how likely was an individual to suffer a heart attack and how likely was that heart attack to be fatal? The results were clear: the conductors had considerably less heart-disease than the drivers. Moreover, when conductors did develop heart-disease, they were likely to do so later in life and the severity of the disease was likely to be less than for the drivers. All in all, the drivers were *twice* as likely to die from a heart attack than the conductors.

The key difference? The drivers sat for most of their work days while the conductors walked and climbed the stairs of their double-decker buses.

The researchers went on to hypothesize possible explanations for the difference. Perhaps men who chose to become conductors were physically stronger than those who chose to become bus drivers. Perhaps being a bus driver was more stressful than being a bus conductor. Ultimately, the researchers rejected these other causes and concluded that the most likely explanation was that "the physical effort in the conductors' work may be a protective factor, safeguarding them in middle age from some of the worst manifestations of heart-disease suffered by less active workers."

The researchers, "interested to see whether the experience of the transport workers were repeated," went on to analyze data from about 110,000 civil servants including postmen, telegraph officers, supervisors, and telephonists. They noted that the postmen were the most active of the group, though their work was "not particularly strenuous" involving "mostly walking, with a variable amount of stair-climbing, cycling, and light carrying." Once again, the results showed that the incidence of heart-disease and related fatality was significantly lower among the more active postmen than among the more sedentary workers.

More walking leads to stronger hearts and lower risk of heart attack and ensuing death. Check. But what happens if you do have a heart attack? Then what?

Exercise and Heart Recovery

Before the bus study and prior to the 1950s, doctors, researchers, and the general public failed to appreciate the value of physical activity to protect our heart health, much less on heart recovery. The past 70 years have seen a seismic shift in our understanding of how to help injured hearts recover.

As recently as the 1940s, patients with heart disease were put on strict bed rest and instructed to move as little as possible for up to six weeks – yup, six weeks of total inactivity. And I mean total. Many were not permitted to feed themselves, as the act of moving fork to mouth was considered potentially dangerous exertion. Bed pans were the norm, as the journey from bed to bathroom was thought to be far too strenuous for a healing heart.

Treatment protocol was predicated on the belief that heart disease was caused by overtaxing the heart and so, the thinking went, the best treatment was to avoid any strain so as to allow the heart to fully rest and recover. This was the prevailing and accepted treatment for decades. It didn't go so well: 35% of those who survived an initial heart attack died while in the hospital and the long-term recovery rates were similarly poor.

We've learned a lot since then. Not only have we developed a far better understanding of the mechanism of heart disease and discovered ways to treat it, we have learned that the heart is a muscle that can be strengthened through exercise. Now, rather than strict bed rest, doctors aim to have cardiac patients up and moving as soon as possible. Many patients are discharged from the hospital and sent to formal cardiac rehabilitation centers. Most are sent home with a formal prescription for an exercise program. Some join walking groups, like those created by Dr. David Sabgir, the cardiologist who founded the not-for-profit "Walk with a Doc."

"Everyday, I would see patients who didn't take their medication and didn't get any exercise." Dr. Sabgir explained when we spoke. "They had all kinds of excuses – they would say *'I would love to get more exercise, but I can't because of my ankle, my knee, my back ...'* They would tell me that they didn't believe that they could do enough exercise for it to matter." Frustrated, Dr. Sabgir decided to try something different and invited patients to walk with him and each other. The approach worked.

Walking as part of a group "enabled us to "attack the problem from multiple angles," Dr. Sabgir told me. "In addition to the powerful physical benefits, walking delivers the mental health benefits that so many of my patients need: the improved self-esteem and reduction in anxiety and depression."

"I remember a woman who came to my practice at over 300 pounds who was very challenged as far as mobility. That first day, she was only able to walk 100 feet, but she stayed with it, slowly building up to a mile and beyond. It was transformative for her." Since then, Dr. Sabgir's Walk with a Doc has spread to other communities with health care professionals leading hundreds of walks and connecting thousands of patients.

Like any muscle, heart strength should be built slowly and over time and of course, if you have any heart disease – or risk of heart disease – any exercise program should only be undertaken with the advice of your doctor. Most will encourage you to get moving.

Walking and Cancer ... Before, During, and After

My Aunt Lee made the very best chocolate mousse. It was incredibly rich and super smooth. Like chocolate mousse meets chocolate pudding. Rumor has it that she used raw egg yolks, but that's just a rumor. One night around the dinner table, my parents told my sister and me that Aunt Lee was sick and there was little the doctors could do. The details were sketchy and it was clear that more info was not going to be forthcoming. She was gone just weeks later. As far as I know, no one ever got her chocolate mousse recipe.

When I was a kid, cancer was the Voldemort of diseases – the disease that must not be named. A cancer diagnosis was something to be whispered. A secret to be hidden as long as possible. This secrecy added to the fear and, I assume, to the isolation of treatment.

But times are a-changin'.

Ceil was the neighbor and best friend of my high school boyfriend's sister. She was a few years older than me; beautiful, spunky, and super-cool in the way that only the super-cool-best-friend-of-your-boyfriend's-older-sister could be. Ceil and I had lost touch for almost two decades, but reconnected as adults on social media. And, from all appearances, she's still super cool. Ceil announced her breast cancer diagnosis with a post on social media with the words "my turn" accompanied by a pink ribbon.

Of course, she's not the only friend I know who has battled breast cancer. Far from it.

I remember the night I met Denise. We were guests at a press dinner and sat next to one another at the end of a long table. We ate truffle fries and talked a mile-a-minute. I describe Denise as nicer than she is beautiful – and if you know Denise, you know that's a very high bar. She shared her diagnosis first with family and friends, and then used her platform as a media personality to share her story and advocate for more compassion, more awareness, and less isolation for other cancer warriors.

During treatment, both of Ceil and Denise's social media feeds were filled with strength, love, and friendship. Both shared images of friends accompanying them to chemo, showed gratitude for their medical teams, and shared posts that made it clear that their lives had not stopped. That yes, #cancersucks, but even in the throes of treatment, the lives they cherish continued. Kids went to camp, dogs played, business grew, plans were made, and treatments were endured.

Both survived. Denise went on to found a not-for-profit dedicated to providing authentic community and meaningful support to other cancer warriors. Ceil went on to years of travel, family, fun, and puppies.

Others, including my friend Alison, whose daughter you will meet shortly, and about 600,000 others each year, do not.

With about 40% of us likely to confront a cancer diagnosis at some point in our lifetime, we should all do what we can to reduce our risk of *getting* cancer and our risk of *dying* from cancer.

Walking can do both.

Walking Reduces Risk

"There is consistent, compelling evidence that physical activity plays a role in preventing many types of cancer and for improving longevity among cancer survivors." In 2020, researchers analyzed nine different studies involving more than 750,000 adults in an effort to determine if their level of physical activity corresponded with the likelihood of them developing cancer. The study found that between 2.5 and 5 hours of moderate-intensity activity or between 1.25 and 2.5 hours of vigorous activity significantly lowered the risk for seven types of cancer including colon, breast, endometrial, kidney, multiple myeloma, liver, and Non-Hodgkin's lymphoma. For several diseases, more exercise correlated with an even greater reduction in the risk.

But what about breast cancer? The most common form of cancer for women, one in eight American women will be diagnosed with breast cancer at some point in her life. There, the researchers concluded that between 2.5 and 5 hours of moderate-intensity activity such as brisk walking reduced the risk of breast cancer by between 6% and 10% and more physical activity reduced that risk further.

While many studies look at the impact of physical activity generally on the risk of breast cancer, Harvard Medical School reported on a study specifically on walking, which revealed that women who walked seven or more hours a week had a 14% lower risk of breast cancer than those who walked three hours or fewer per week.

Yet another study sought to ascertain if even those women with a genetic predisposition to breast cancer would benefit from a regular walking practice. This study concluded that 2.7 weekly hours of moderate exercise such as walking was associated with a 20% lower breast cancer risk.

More walking. Less cancer. Check.

Walking Improves Likelihood of Survival

A regular walking practice can reduce your risk of developing several types of cancer. But what happens after you get that terrifying call? Once diagnosed, is it time to hang up your walking shoes until treatment is concluded? If you made that choice, you wouldn't be alone as studies have noted that many cancer patients decrease activity or become inactive during or after treatment.

It would seem to make sense to assume that your body needs all of its energy reserves to handle treatment and combat the disease. Why else would you feel so deeply exhausted?

Yet research strongly suggests otherwise. A significant study published in 2020 dove deep into the impact of physical activity before, during, and after chemotherapy and the relationship between physical activity, cancer recurrence, and likelihood of survival. The results were striking: those who reported the highest levels of physical activity before they were diagnosed reduced their risk of death by 26% to 27%.

The impact becomes even greater with those who maintain – or even increase – their activity during treatment. Those breast cancer warriors who maintained the highest levels of activity *following* diagnosis showed even stronger protection, reducing the risk of death by 39% to 48% as compared to those who were least active.

And following treatment? Preliminary research suggests that exercise may reduce the risk of a recurrence. The researchers observed:

- High-risk breast cancer patients who engaged in at least 150 minutes of moderate-intensity physical activity each week both before and *after* diagnosis experienced greater than 50% reduced risk of recurrence and mortality compared with those who did not;
- Patients who did not engage in at least 150 minutes of weekly physical activity *prior* to diagnosis but did so *after* treatment experienced statistically significant reduced risk of recurrence and mortality.

Why? How?

The researchers noted several possible mechanisms by which exercise reduces cancer risk including the regulation of body fat, the effects of physical activity on estrogen metabolism, insulin sensitivity, chronic inflammation, oxidative stress, or immune function. Maybe it improves the way the body puts chemotherapy to work. Perhaps there are benefits from the mental and emotional upsides of walking – such as those we discussed before – reduced stress, improved mood, better ability to process challenges, and more awe. Maybe it is all these things, or some combination of these things. Or maybe it is something else. However it happens, study after study shows that it does.

For Alison Webster, maintaining her walking practice throughout her battle with metastatic breast cancer was key to helping her feel as healthy and strong as possible for as long as possible. "Her walking practice did so much for her," her daughter Katie shared with me one winter morning.

"She would set monthly walking goals, but didn't care if she met them or not, as long as she did something every day. She taught me that small steps still count and forward momentum is what matters."

Sometimes, they walked together by the river. "I'd been having a rough time, and wanted to turn back. But there were a series of benches along the way and mum would say, *'Let's just get to the next bench,'* and then the next, and the next, until we got to her favorite. Then we'd sit together for a while."

Small steps count and forward momentum is what matters.

Sugar Rush: Walking and Diabetes

If we are going to continue working our way down the list of deadly diseases that can be ameliorated by walking, let's next consider Type 2 diabetes, high on the list of preventable diseases that kills millions of people worldwide each year. According to the Mayo Clinic, "the prevalence of diabetes is increasing at an alarming rate not only in the United States but also worldwide."

Behind diabetes is insulin misregulation. Insulin is a hormone produced in the pancreas that enables our body to use the food we eat to provide the energy we need. Insulin is also pressed into service to help store energy that we might need for later, perhaps in between meals or at times of stress. If your body becomes resistant to insulin, it may begin to overproduce it in an effort to keep your blood glucose levels normal. Over time, this can impair the function of your pancreas and result in Type 2 diabetes.

You know what helps? Walking.

Walking Can Help Prevent Type-2 Diabetes

It's not like we don't know the risk factors for Type 2 diabetes, which include elevated blood sugar levels, being overweight, and leading a sedentary lifestyle. In many cases, doctors can see the markers for the potential for Type 2 diabetes long before the disease takes hold.

In a study published in the New England Journal of Medicine, researchers set out to discover if lifestyle interventions could be as effective as medication in preventing or delaying the onset of diabetes for an at-risk population. Turns out, they were more effective.

Noting that Type 2 diabetes is a "serious, costly disease affecting approximately 8% of adults in the United States" for which current treatment methods are "inadequate," the team set out to answer the following questions: "Can lifestyle changes or treatment with medication prevent or delay the onset of diabetes? Which one is better? Does their effectiveness differ according to age, sex, or race or ethnic group?"

3,234 individuals who were at risk of developing diabetes were randomly assigned to one of three groups:

- Group One was provided with standard lifestyle recommendations, which included written information and an annual individual session which emphasized the importance of a healthy lifestyle and encouraged them to reduce their weight and increase their physical activity. Group One was also prescribed daily medication which has been shown to reduce diabetes risk;

- Group Two was provided with the same standard lifestyle recommendations, but instead of daily preventive medication, Group Two was given a placebo;

- Group Three was provided with an "intensive lifestyle intervention" that included being encouraged to adopt a healthy low-calorie, low-fat diet and to engage in physical activity of moderate intensity, such as brisk walking, for at least 150 minutes per week. They were provided ongoing education and given individual support for 24 weeks. They were not given medication or placebo.

When the researchers checked in with the study participants more than two-and-a-half years later, those who had participated in the intensive lifestyle intervention reduced their incidence of developing diabetes by 58%, while the group that took medication reduced their incidence of developing diabetes by merely 31%. Notably, the study did not show that walking alone was responsible for this dramatic reduction in diabetes risk, but rather physical activity was an integral part of lifestyle changes that included improved diet, reduced weight, and increased physical activity. But that combination proved to be highly-effective – more effective than medication.

Improved diet and more movement equals less diabetes. Check.

For the Sake of Your Blood Sugar, Does it Matter When You Walk?

When I was 23, my parents sold our family home and moved to Florida. I wasn't happy about it, but they bought a beautiful house in a great family neighborhood. There were kids riding bikes and always someone with whom to play tennis. I visited often and whenever I did, we fell into a routine of taking an after-dinner walk together around the two-mile perimeter of the community. I always thought of it as time to talk and enjoy the unique feel of the warm Florida evening air against my skin.

But that wasn't all we were doing on those walks. We were also leveling out our blood sugar in a way that was really good for our bodies.

Researchers continue to investigate how much physical activity – and when – is most protective and effective at regulating blood-sugar levels. A recent study compared the effect of a 45-minute daily walk with three 15-minute walks, one following each meal. The study suggests that 15 minutes of walking done 30 minutes after each meal was equally effective as 45 minutes of sustained morning walking and significantly lowered blood sugar levels. Notably, the exertion level of these 15 minute walks were "barely of moderate intensity, suggesting that the timing of exercise may be as important (if not more) as volume and intensity in determining the best exercise prescriptions for glycemic control in older people."

Lose Weight

What Diet Culture Has Done to Us

There is no question that diet culture has done a tremendous disservice to us all. For decades, we have been offered a litany of diets – some crazy and some not so crazy – as a solution to our ever-increasing girth and the many lifestyle and health challenges that accompany it. The cabbage soup diet. The grapefruit diet. The lemonade diet. The baby food diet (yup, that's a thing). We have been sold an astounding assortment of teas, elixirs, and drugs under the auspices of weight loss promises. We have been shamed, cajoled, and threatened with headlines that have convinced us that we are less than if our weight is more than.

Before we explore the power of walking for weight management, let me first remind you that you are not the number on the scale, the circumference of your waist, or your dress size. You will never be able to hate yourself healthy.

However, there are very real health consequences that result from carrying extra weight, and even more that come from tipping the scale to obesity. You don't need me to tell you that – we have all heard it more times than we care to count.

And there is no one single thing that will instantly melt 20, 30, 50 or 100 pounds from your frame. There is no magic bullet or secret potion. But there are lifestyle changes that, over time, and for most of us – barring any unusual medical condition that impacts the way you process and use food – can help you achieve and maintain a weight that enables you to function at your best.

Walking is one of those lifestyle changes.

There's More To It Than Calories In and Calories Out

I was sitting at work one morning when I received an email from a guy who was building an app he claimed better calculated the calories consumed in the food you eat and expended by the exercise you do. He was asking for my advice and it sounded like he had an innovative idea, so we scheduled a call. It didn't go well.

"Accurately figuring out exactly how many calories people are eating is the single key to helping people lose weight and beating the obesity crisis," he argued. "People need better data." He is not alone. Many believe that weight loss and weight management is a simple mathematical equation: calories in versus calories out.

While there is a basic truth to that, the reality is far, far more complex. *First*, physiologically, we all process foods in different ways. Our systems work differently. *Second*, not every calorie is created equal as far as how it impacts our minds, moods, and bodies. *And finally*, and perhaps most importantly, there are mental, habitual, societal, cultural, and emotional elements that impact how we eat and how we move.

I'm not convinced that we simply need more data. But I am convinced that a regular walking practice can be an extremely powerful tool for reasons that are as complex as the weight-loss challenge itself.

Sure, walking burns calories and that is essential to any weight loss journey. But walking offers so much more. The food we eat is connected to how we feel, how we've been socialized, and what we believe. It is how many of us manage stress and anxiety. It is how we celebrate and how we mourn. We self-medicate our depression with donuts. We find companionship in cookies. We feed our low self-worth with sweet tea.

It is all connected.

Walking boosts our mood and helps clear the cobwebs. Walking offers an outlet to help process our emotions. Walking with others connects us in a profound and powerful way. Walking shows us that we can move forward, and convinces us that we have the strength and the fortitude to take steps towards better. Walking helps us sleep better and poor sleep is connected with weight gain and obesity.

Walking connects you with your body and better enables you to hear its cues. Walking helps manage stress and reduces cortisol levels and increased stress and increased cortisol have also been linked to obesity. As we've seen, walking helps regulate blood sugar levels and makes you happier.

And ...

Yup, Walking Burns Calories

I know I shared my frustration with the guy who believes that better calorie data is *the* answer to all weight loss challenges. It's not. But calories in and calories out does matter.

How many calories you will expend on a walk depends on a host of factors, but just to offer a baseline *estimate* (emphasis on estimate), a woman who weighs 150 pounds will burn approximately 200 calories an hour walking at a moderate pace. Several factors impact this including your fitness level, the efficiency with which your body works, the terrain on which you walk, the temperature, and your unique physiology. But one thing is clear: walking burns calories.

Enough to make a difference? This study says yes.

A team of researchers set out to answer a pretty basic question: how much physical activity is necessary to impact body weight and composition of individuals who are overweight or have mild obesity? The researchers randomized 120 men and women between the ages of 40 and 65 who were told that they were participating in an exercise – not a weight loss – study and were instructed not to diet or alter their daily caloric intake.

They were then randomly divided into four groups:

- Group One exercised the equivalent of walking or jogging about 11 miles/week at an average pace of about 16-minutes per mile;
- Group Two exercised the equivalent of walking or jogging 11 miles/week at an average pace of about 10-minutes per mile;
- Group Three exercised the equivalent of walking or jogging about 17 miles/week at an average pace of about 10-minutes per mile;
- Group Four was the control group that did not engage in any additional physical activity.

At the end of eight months, the researchers concluded that there is a "clear dose-response relationship between the amount of exercise and the amount of weight change," despite the fact that there had been no significant changes to the participants' diets and no calorie restriction. Specifically:

- Group One lost an average of 2.9 lbs;
- Group Two lost an average of 2.4 lbs;
- Group Three lost an average of 7.7 lbs; and
- The Control Group gained an average of 2.4 lbs.

Though any meaningful weight loss plan should include a combination of nutrition and exercise, more walking is definitely a step in the right direction.

She Tried Everything.

To meet Andrea Heuston before 2007 would have been to meet a professional woman who had it all together. Career. Family. Home. By all measures, she was incredibly successful. "But the one place I felt completely out of control was my weight. No matter what I did," Andrea confided during one of our several conversations about her walking and weight loss journey, "I couldn't lose weight." Her desperation to assert control over her weight almost cost her her life.

"I tried every diet I could find. Nothing worked. In 2007, I opted for lap-band surgery." Lab-band surgery is an invasive, bariatric surgery in which a band is placed around your stomach to reduce its capacity, with the goal of making you feel more full with less food. While many have had success with this procedure, many have not. One 2014 study reported that 44% of the study's participants' lap-band surgeries failed for one reason or another.

For Andrea, lap-band surgery was a disaster, with complication after complication, the last of which landed her in a coma. For 17 days. "When I woke up, I knew I had to take control of my health." She began walking. Slowly at first, as she recovered from the coma and regained her strength. Bit by bit, Andrea added steps and increased her daily mileage. "Now," she says, "I typically take 20,000 steps a day, though I recently stopped counting because I realize I can get a little obsessive."

The benefits of Andrea's walking practice have gone far beyond her getting control of her weight and health, though that is what prompted her walking journey. "What walking does for me is not just help me maintain a healthy weight, it helps me stay sane," she explains. "A walk can reset my mood when I'm feeling tense or anxious, and give me the time and space to think creatively and strategically." And Andrea has added a social component to her walking practice. "Every Saturday, I walk with a group of women I went to high school with. We have created a bond – a friendship – that I didn't know I'd be able to have at this stage of my life."

Stress management. Connection with her body. Social bonds. Time away from screens. And the ability, finally, to maintain a healthy weight.

Eat Less Chocolate

You know the feeling. At least, I know the feeling. I walk in the door after a long and stressful day, drop my keys in the key bowl, and head to the pantry. And there they are: those delicious little nuggets of dark chocolate. I tell myself that just a few will satisfy the craving. But one becomes two and two becomes four and, at some point, all those little nuggets become the equivalent of a full-sized Snickers.

Ah, chocolate cravings. For many, chocolate represents one of the strongest food cravings. Why? Other than the fact that chocolate is typically high in sugar and fat – a combination that we humans are wired to crave – no one is exactly sure why many crave chocolate over, say, equally sweet and fat-laden vanilla pudding. There is some evidence that eating chocolate releases the feel-good hormone dopamine. Chocolate, at least good quality dark chocolate, can also be a source of magnesium, a key nutrient that many Americans – women in particular – tend to be deficient in. Finally, chocolate, or the cacao on which it is based, contains many other compounds and so perhaps there is some magic, feel-good chemical hidden in that chocolate bar that we have yet to identify.

Regardless of why, once that chocolate craving hits, it can be hard to fight. So if walking can help tamp down a seemingly all-powerful chocolate craving, imagine what it could do for other cravings which, for many of us, are not quite as compelling as that jar of chocolate nuggets in the pantry.

Turns out, it can. Studies have shown that a single, 15-minute brisk walk can materially reduce the urge to eat chocolate, even among regular chocolate eaters who have been exposed to a stressful situation. This decrease in the craving for chocolatey, sugary, yummy snacks following a 15-minute walk works even for people who have a propensity for sugary snacks and struggle with their weight.

It's not just chocolate. Merely ten minutes of moderate exercise can help reduce nicotine cravings among smokers.

If a walk can help derail chocolate and nicotine cravings, chances are good that it can help derail other cravings for unhealthy things.

I know that it worked for me. When I was a college sophomore craving something that was not aligned with my goal of walking off the freshman 30, I would often make a deal with myself. If, after a two-mile walk I still wanted it, I would have it. More often than not, I would return from that walk and the craving was gone or, if not gone, at least it had abated enough that I was able to ignore it.

Oh, My Aching Back: Walking and Back Pain

My mother was a professional dancer with what she often referred to as a "bad back." She'd be fine for months, kicking, spinning, and Martha-Grahaming in front of the big picture window in our living room that doubled as a mirror at night, heading off to rehearsals, performing here, there, and everywhere. Until she "threw out her back," which was rarely the result of a too-high kick, and more often the result of "getting out of bed wrong."

Now, of course, getting out of bed wrong was merely the last straw of cumulative damage, but it is often the silly, household movements that are the ultimate trigger: picking up the laundry basket, twisting to get out of the car, emptying the dishwasher.

When my mother's back would go out, she would take to her bed in misery and lie as still as possible. Occasionally, it would be so bad that the doctor would arrive, old-fashioned black bag in hand, and inject muscle relaxants into her spasmed back. She would remain prone, until the worst of it passed, slowly easing back into life and movement.

Fast forward 50 years and my mother, now in her mid-80s, still wrestles with a "bad back" including pain that radiates from her back down her legs. A recent MRI showed an unhappy disc. "The doctor said if I was younger, he'd go in and clean it up," she explained after her most recent appointment. "But at 86, I think I'm just going to live with it."

"What's the plan for how to do that?" I asked.

"I'm just going to keep walking. Every day, I'm going to do what I can."

She's right.

Back pain can be caused by many different things. An inflamed, bulging, or heaven-forbid ruptured disc. A pinched nerve. Muscle strains in everything from your erector muscles to your traps to your psoas. Pelvic floor issues. Posture issues. Too much time sitting. A desk that is too high or too low. Osteoporosis. Osteoarthritis. The list of back pain culprits is very, very long.

Back pain can also be caused by problems with your kidneys or endometriosis or several other more serious problems that don't originate in your back, even though that might be where you feel it most. Meaning, if you have back pain, it is important to have it checked out. But once it is clear that your back pain is being caused by a run-of-the-mill issue and your doctor has cleared you to move – take a walk.

In 2017, a group of researchers analyzed nine different studies that considered the benefits of walking on pain, disability, and quality of life in connection with chronic lower back pain. They began by noting that research has shown that a variety of exercise programs benefit people with chronic back pain, including muscle strengthening, flexibility, and aerobic training, but that up to 70% of people who start an exercise program abandon it.

The researchers sought to determine if walking, what they referred to as a "fundamental human activity" with low barriers, low risk of injury, and high overall health benefits, would prove to be as good for chronic lower back pain as other more complicated exercise programs.

It was.

Though the researchers noted that additional research could be beneficial, they concluded that the evidence showed that walking was as effective as other non-pharmacological interventions (e.g. exercise, education, or physiotherapy) in terms of "pain and disability reduction" and that those benefits lasted for three to twelve months.

Two caveats: if walking makes the pain flare up or get worse, don't do it. If you have no idea what is causing your back pain, find out.

Oh My Aching Knees: Walking and Arthritis

Some mornings, I feel this weird tenderness in the joint of my big toe. It's not severe and I can totally ignore it, but it got me wondering. Could it be arthritis? Can you get arthritis in your toes?

Apparently you can.

Arthritis is swelling and tenderness in your joints which can cause pain and stiffness ranging from "hmmmm, that feels a little achy" to utterly debilitating. It can appear in any joint – including your toes – but tends to be especially noticeable – and problematic – in the knees, hips, hands, back, and feet.

If I am beginning to suffer the effects of arthritis, I'm not alone. The CDC estimates that 24% of all adults, or 58.5 million people in the US alone, have arthritis.

There are several types and causes of arthritis, including osteoarthritis, Rheumatoid Arthritis, Lupus, Psoriatic arthritis, gout, and others. Importantly, the triggers and treatments differ among the type of arthritis and the individual: what helps one person might not help another and if you are experiencing joint pain – especially pain that is worsening – it is time to see a medical professional to understand what is going on.

Osteoarthritis is the most common and is often called the "wear and tear" arthritis. However, researcher and professor of medicine Dr. Grace Hsiao-Wei Lo is quick to point out that "most researchers who study this disease, including me, do not like the term 'wear and tear' arthritis because it suggests that no matter what you do, if you use your joints, they will deteriorate. This is not the case. Although age is a substantial risk factor for the disease, not everyone who ages gets osteoarthritis. We can make choices that can modify our risk of developing symptoms and having worsening structure."

Among those choices? Walking.

Dr. Lo led a study that investigated the impact of a regular walking practice on more than 1,000 individuals who were showing signs of osteoarthritis in their knees. The study followed them for four years and found that those who walked for exercise were 40% less likely to develop regular knee pain compared to those who did not walk for exercise. The results also suggested those individuals who walked for exercise were less likely to have worsening of the severity of their arthritis. "These are important findings," Dr. Lo explains, "because they suggest walking can perhaps be a treatment that influences *both* symptoms and structure in osteoarthritis. If so, this would be the first treatment that would offer both. It also suggests that perhaps our focus on medications to treat osteoarthritis might need to be broadened to really focus on the biomechanical aspects of the condition."

For 63-year-old Marsha Whisnant, who suffers from osteoarthritis in both knees, walking was a game-changer. A widow, mother to two, and grandmother to five, Marsha was diagnosed with osteoarthritis several years ago "when it got to the point that walking was very painful." A physician advised Marsha that the best thing she could do was start walking. It wasn't easy. "When I first started, walking hurt. I couldn't go fast or far, but I kept at it and everything improved. I lost weight, the pain became much less, and I was finally able to walk without limping." Marsha built up to more than three miles and walks early most mornings before work. Her walking practice has kept her arthritis pain at bay and given her back the opportunity to enjoy her kids and grandkids. "To call walking a game-changer is like calling the Grand Canyon a ditch."

Remember, as with all new walking programs, consult your medical professional to be sure it is safe for you to start a new program and be like Marsha: start slowly, build slowly, and keep going.

Stronger Bones

"Doc," I whined (even at 57, I wasn't beyond the occasional whine), "I've done everything right."

"You'd be in much worse shape if you hadn't," explained the doctor with the Sean Connery accent.

It was my follow-up appointment with the director of osteoporosis at a prestigious New York hospital. He was trying to explain how it was that I, who had discovered walking at 16 and weightlifting at 18 – and haven't stopped either since – was suffering from rapidly-progressing osteopenia, the precursor to osteoporosis. My bone density wasn't terrible – yet – but at 57, I was heading in the wrong direction and fast.

We tend to think of our bones as fixed and solid, like the metal scaffolding of the skyscraper of our bodies. But that's not true. Our bones are constantly breaking down and rebuilding themselves, replacing old, worn-out tissue with new, fresh, strong bone. Sometimes, that equation gets out of whack and more bone gets broken down than gets rebuilt. The result?

Osteopenia and osteoporosis, which can lead to fractures, disability, and, ultimately, death.

Osteoporosis is no joke.

Among the biggest culprits in causing osteoporosis? Age. Being female. Going through menopause. So yeah, life.

One of the best ways to help keep osteoporosis and the potential for fractures at bay?

Walking.

Build Your Bones Before Menopause

Let's begin by going back in time. Since some bone loss is inevitable as we age, a key to combating osteoporosis later in life is to maximize bone density earlier in life. Starting when you are young – particularly during adolescence and our early 20s – it is important to eat a healthy diet and get lots of physical activity, including resistance, weight bearing, and impact. Walk, run, jump, play, and pick up and put down heavy things.

Continue that good diet and physical activity throughout your life.

Then, in the years leading up to menopause, walk. A study of 222 women between the ages of 45 and 50 who had not yet gone through menopause showed that two years of a regular "brisk" walking practice had a "positive effect" on bone density.

Keep Going After Menopause

What about after menopause, when bone loss appears to be tied directly to the drop in women's estrogen levels? Here, the effects of walking on bone density have been widely considered with somewhat inconsistent results. However, the prevailing evidence supports the conclusion that walking can help maintain bone density levels and prevent or slow bone loss, depending on the individual as well as the intensity, consistency, and duration of her practice. Add some hills and some stairs and all the better.

As one study showed, "healthy postmenopausal women who walk approximately one-mile each day have higher whole-body bone density than women who walk shorter distances. Walking is also effective in slowing the rate of bone loss from the legs. These results strongly support the widely-held belief that walking is a beneficial form of physical activity for maintaining skeletal integrity."

What of the studies that suggest walking doesn't help? In a study that showed two years of brisk walking has positive effects on bone density, the researchers speculated that perhaps the inconsistency of prior studies is the result of their short intervention period because bone metabolism is a slow process that can take 12 months or longer before a new steady state of bone metabolism can be reached.

What About the Men?

Sorry, guys, but osteoporosis is not just a girl-thing. Though the post-menopausal decline in bone density is more sudden and more pronounced in women, the reality is that men's bones also weaken as they age. In fact, by the time men are in their mid-60s, many are losing bone at the same rate as women.

According to the Bone Health & Osteoporosis Foundation:

- Up to one in four men over age 50 will break a bone due to osteoporosis;
- Approximately two million American men already have osteoporosis and about 12 million more are at risk;
- Men older than 50 are more likely to break a bone due to osteoporosis than they are to get prostate cancer;
- Each year, about 80,000 men will break a hip.

Despite these statistics, most men consider osteoporosis a "women's disease." Few doctors consider bone health for their male patients and few men are proactive about protecting their bone health. But they should be.

Bone Density Doesn't Tell the Whole Story

As my personal experience shows, walking might not be enough to over-come a strong genetic propensity for osteoporosis or any one of a dozen other things that can lead to bone loss. Nevertheless, there is sufficient evidence to show that it helps.

Moreover, the risk of osteoporosis is not simply that your bones become weaker: having less-dense bones is only problematic if you break them. That's why most osteoporosis specialists don't just look at bone density, they consider additional factors in an effort to more accurately assess frac-ture risk. Those factors include your medical history, other medical prob-lems, your weight ... even how much alcohol and coffee you drink.

And there's more. How's your balance? How strong are your muscles? How likely are you to fall?

All of those things are helped by a regular walking practice.

More walking, stronger muscles, and less falling. Less falling, less fracturing.

There is one more key to preventing falls and ensuing fractures: better balance.

Better Balance

I was tired. I had been traveling. Perhaps I was dehydrated or congested or maybe the altitude was getting to me. But as I walked down the hallway of the Park City hotel, the floor tilted and threw me against the wall. I stood there for a few minutes, hoping the floor would return to its usual flat and stable position. It was a bout of vertigo, brought on by who knows what. My balance returned as the morning went on and that disconcerting feeling hasn't returned since, but I vividly remember the disorienting walk down that hotel hallway.

Balance is something we take for granted. Until we lose it.

Maintaining our balance is the result of a remarkable and complex system. It begins with the vestibular system located inside the inner ear which is comprised of canals, organs filled with fluid and tiny, sensitive hairs. When our head moves, the fluid shifts, touching the hairs and sending feedback to the brain, which then, almost instantaneously, processes and dispatches that information, instructing the rest of our body to execute the many micro-adjustments needed to navigate the curb, react to a slip, or continue walking upright as we lift our chin to catch a snowflake on our tongue. At the same time, our eyes process everything from the height of the curb and our bodies send additional data about the patch of ice as we begin to slip.

The almost magical complexity of balance is the reason why we have sent telescopes into space that are strong enough to view the beginning of the universe yet have not managed to make a robot that can walk as gracefully as a human being (though as of this writing, we are getting closer).

As we age, the integrated systems that enable us to maintain our balance begin to deteriorate. Our brains don't process as quickly and our muscles don't respond as quickly, either. If we do fall, the consequences can be worse, as those slower reflexes reduce our ability to catch ourselves. And, to make matters even worse, if we do hit the ground, weaker bones are more likely to fracture.

And here's the rub: a Duke University study of 775 adults showed that balance begins to decline in the 50s with other studies suggesting balance decline might begin even earlier.

Poor balance has significant potential health consequences. The CDC reports that about 36 million falls are reported among older adults each year, resulting in more than 3 million emergency room visits and more than 32,000 deaths. And while not all falls can be prevented, maintaining strength and balance can help.

In 2015, a team of researchers from Japan sought to determine whether or not a walking program reduced the risk of falling for older adults. The question is complicated by the fact that more walking presents more opportunities for falling: if you rarely move from the couch, you rarely have an opportunity to fall. The researchers explained it this way: "The problematic nature of a walking intervention aimed at fall prevention is that along with the improvement in physical and psychological functions, it is also accompanied by increased exposure to environmental hazards (e.g., a greater chance of tripping while walking)." To account for this, the researchers sought to measure the likelihood that a trip would result in a fall.

The study included 90 adults ages 65 to 79 who did not exhibit anything that put them at a higher fall risk – no injuries, limited medication, and no history of recent falls. The participants were broken into two groups. Both groups engaged in a 12-week program that included lectures, a warm up, a recreational activity, the primary exercise, and a cool down. For the exercise portion, the "walking group" walked briskly on a pedestrian road, while the "balance training group" engaged in a program that included strength training and Tai Chi (long considered an effective balance training modality). Both groups were instructed to continue their exercise routines at home and record any incidence of trips or falls for the following year. The result? The walking group showed a "significant reduction" in the risk of falling.

The researchers considered possible explanations for why the walking intervention improved balance and reduced fall risk.

First, the walking protocol helped to build the participants' endurance, and the researchers noted that a person is more likely to fall when they are fatigued. Thus, improved endurance could help prevent falls.

Second, the walking group experienced significantly more trips than the balance group did. At first, this might seem to be a negative. But the researchers noted that the quick initiation of a recovery step after a trip is key to avoiding a fall. In other words, tripping practice could have an "inoculating effect" on the likelihood that a trip results in a fall.

Then there's the possibility that the walking program helps to prevent what Doctor of Physical Therapy Meghan Griech refers to as the downward spiral. "Strength is essential for balance," she explained to me. "Often, I see a spiral of decline in my patients," she said. "They suffer a fall or an injury, they become fearful and reduce the amount they walk. Less walking leads to a deterioration in the physical strength needed to respond and adapt, causing more fear, which in turn leads to less walking. This negative cycle can be slow and insidious," she cautions. "I tell all of my patients, 'as long as you feel stable in your joints, you need to walk every day, preferably several times each day.'"

Menopause is Sneaky. Walking Helps.

For decades, I would brush my teeth, wash my face, and take a low-dose hormone birth control pill. I had two kids, one of whom I gave birth to the old-fashioned way and the other adopted when she was 10-months old. Our family was complete, built in just the way I had always dreamed – from the time I was a little girl, I always said I was going to have a baby and adopt a baby.

One night, somewhere in my mid-40s, I took a look at the pill just before popping it in my mouth and thought, *"Hmmmm, I've been taking these for the better part of 20 years. That seems like a long time to be putting artificial hormones in my body."*

The next morning, I shared my feelings with my husband who replied, "Well, you've been taking responsibility for this for our entire relationship. I suppose it is my turn." He offered to get a vasectomy.

I stopped taking the pill and plans were made.

Within days, my sleep, always reliable and vital to my well-being in every way, was completely disrupted. Night sweats. Insomnia. Anxiety. Mood swings.

I was a mess.

Several weeks passed before one of my best childhood friends and his wife came to visit for the weekend. Over early morning coffee, I told him what was going on. I hadn't exactly connected my new-found insomnia and other symptoms with stopping the pill cold turkey, but he did.

"You are young, healthy, never smoked, and have no history of cancer in your family," he said. "Go back on the pill until you're 50," he advised.

My husband happily canceled his appointment and I refilled my prescription. Within days, I was myself again. Though I am not recommending that you use birth control pills as a form of hormone replacement therapy (I have since learned that this is not a great plan), my experience showed me, in a dramatic fashion, the impact of perimenopause on practically every one of my body's systems.

Perimenopause is sneaky, delivering a myriad of unique and personal symptoms ranging from sleep disruption, brain fog, irregular periods, thinning hair, mood swings, irritability, anxiety, memory lapses, difficulty concentrating, reduced libido, vaginal dryness, fatigue, headaches, and – well, the list of potential impacts from the tremendous hormone fluctuations is varied, individual, and long.

According to Dr. Arianna Sholes-Douglas, a gynecologist and author specializing in menopause, researchers have identified more than 34 symptoms associated with perimenopause and menopause.

While until recently, the topic was largely ignored by the male-dominated medical establishment, things are improving with new studies, new research, new medical specialties, and entire books addressing the symptoms and management of this female rite of passage. We are a long way from understanding menopause in its entirety and the journey is different for everyone, but one thing appears to be true: walking helps.

Here's what we know. Walking helps us regulate sleep, boost mood, ease anxiety, improve memory, manage weight, strengthen bones, and encourage brains to work at their best – all things typically disrupted by perimenopause.

The evidence continues to mount specifically focused on women and menopause. In one study, researchers recruited 190 women between the ages of 40 and 60 who were menopausal or perimenopausal. The women were divided into two groups: the first group undertook a 12-week walking program in which they walked three times each week for three months, building up the pace and duration from 30 minutes to an hour as the weeks progressed. The second group did not engage in any walking or exercise program.

The results were compelling and showed a convincing reduction in a host of menopause symptoms including hot flashes, heart discomfort, sleep problems, depressive mood, irritability, anxiety, exhaustion, sexual problems, bladder problems, vaginal dryness, and joint discomfort.

The researchers concluded that the study revealed "a statistically significant reduction in the frequency and severity of menopausal symptoms."

Get Sick Less

The entire time I was growing up, I don't recall my dad ever being sick. Not one cold, not one flu, not a single stomach bug. That might be the distorted memory of a daughter who was convinced her dad was Superman, but I don't think so. Dad always attributed his extraordinary immune system to two things: his constant exposure to kids and their germs (remember, he was a phys ed teacher and coach) and his regular habit of washing his hands after every class he taught and before every meal he ate. But I'm not so sure. My research suggests that maybe it had more to do with his lifetime of exercise.

While the research on the impact of exercise to help support your immune system is evolving, the evidence is clear: consistent, moderate exercise makes you better able to avoid getting sick and, if you do get sick, helps speed your recovery and reduce your risk of death. How much better? In a paper analyzing more than 20 studies on the connection between exercise and immune response, the authors concluded that the number of days that an individual had an upper respiratory infection was 43% lower for people who averaged five days or more of weekly aerobic exercise. They concluded that "the randomized clinical trials ... are consistent in demonstrating that participants assigned to moderate exercise programs experience reduced upper respiratory infection incidence and duration [the magnitude of which] exceeds levels reported for most medications and supplements."

Walking. Better than medication and supplements.

How? Once again, researchers aren't certain, as our immune system is mind-bendingly complex (at least for me). But appears we can thank a host of impacts including a boost in white blood cells, reduction in inflammation, activation of our lymphatic system, and much more.

Bottom line? More walking equals fewer sick days.

Protect Your Peepers

I had perfect vision my entire life. I threaded every needle with confidence and crushed every eye test. 20/20. When I turned 42, things changed and they changed fast. Forget sticking a piece of thread through the eye of a needle, simply reading for more than ten minutes gave me a piercing headache. The eye doctor nodded knowingly while I lamented the rapid deterioration of my precious eyesight and reassured me when I proclaimed, panicked, that if my eyesight continued to deteriorate at the current rate, it would be entirely gone within just a couple of years.

"Don't worry," he said, "it will stabilize." He prescribed glasses, admonished me to protect my eyes from further sun damage with large, high-quality sunglasses, and sent me on my way.

He was right. My vision did stabilize. I tucked drugstore reading glasses in every nook and cranny of my house, filled a prescription for distance and invested in an expensive pair of progressives for the rest of my daily life. I became protective of my vision, wore sunglasses most of the time, and began to research what, if anything, I could do to help support my vision.

Fast forward a dozen years, and the news got worse. "You have narrow angle glaucoma," that same doctor said on what I had anticipated would be a routine appointment. One of the many types of glaucoma that can result in blindness, narrow-angle glaucoma occurs when the shape of your eyes changes. It's terrifying.

Glaucoma actually includes several different eye conditions, but all have the same resultant risk: pressure in your eye causes damage to your optic nerve. These are very serious conditions that absolutely, positively, require consultation with a qualified and skilled ophthalmologist. Do. Not. Mess. Around.

While only your glaucoma specialist can determine if you have the type of glaucoma that would benefit from exercise, studies have shown that increased levels of physical activity may be associated with decreased odds of developing glaucoma and may prevent the progression in those already diagnosed. And I'm all for stacking the deck to maintain my vision.

But Wait, Is It Exercise That Helps Or Do Healthier People Just Move More?

There is an important difference between correlation and causation. Causation between two events means that one causes the second to occur. For instance, perhaps a study showed that those who drink their coffee with sugar are more likely to need a root canal in the next three years. It would be tempting to draw the conclusion that drinking the sweetened coffee caused the tooth infection that required the root canal. But perhaps, deeper digging would reveal that those who drop a tablespoon of sugar in their morning brew are more likely to also eat more sugar throughout the day, skip their evening tooth cleaning, or something else. Perhaps there is correlation, but not causation.

Correlation between two events means that the two are related in some way, but A does not necessarily cause B to happen. Taking the example above, if you could account for all other variables – meaning the needed-a-root-canal group and the didn't-need-a-root-canal group were identical in all other ways besides how they drank their coffee, you'd get far, far closer to proving causation.

Yup, it's tricky.

For our purposes, the key question is whether exercise *causes* improved health and increases longevity, or is there simply a *correlation* between exercise, health, and longevity. Perhaps it is simply that healthier people tend to move more. This is a question researchers have sought to untangle for years and the evidence continues to mount that, yup, it's the exercise that causes the improved health, wellness, and happiness.

A Finnish study involving nearly 16,000 same-sex twins provides meaningful insight. The study kicked off in 1974 and over the following two decades, researchers surveyed the twins in an effort to determine, among other things, whether it was the genes or the exercise that contributed to improved health and longevity. The researchers classified the participants into three categories:

- "Conditioning Exercisers" included those who exercised at least six times per month at an intensity corresponding to at least a vigorous walk for at least 30 minutes;

- "Sedentary" included those who engaged in no leisure physical activity; and
- "Occasional Exercisers" included everyone else.

20 years later, 1,253 of the participants had died and the researchers were able to take a good look at the impact of exercise on the mortality rates. Even after accounting for other risk factors, exercise proved strongly protective, reducing the death rate of "Conditioning Exercisers" by 43% and "Occasional Exercisers" by 29%.

But was the protection genetic or kinetic? Even among genetically similar twins, exercise was a strong independent predictor of survival. Twins who exercised regularly were 56% less likely to die during the study period than their sedentary siblings, and those twins who exercised only occasionally had a 34% lower death rate than their sedentary siblings.

Thousands of other studies have shown the relationship between exercise in general – and walking in particular – on health, wellness, and longevity. While many factors play a role in the quality and length of our lives, the evidence is clear that walking is a way we can take action to improve our health, well-being and longevity.

Part II: How to Walk

How to Walk

Chances are you've been walking since you were somewhere between 8 and 18 months old. For most of us, that means we've been walking for a long, long time.

Do you really need advice on how to walk?

Probably. Walking is surprisingly complex. It requires the perfect harmony of brain function and muscle coordination. Understanding the mechanics and practicing good form can help you get the most out of every walk and avoid injury.

Moreover, with all of the benefits of walking for your mind, mood, and body, you'd think that pretty much everyone would be doing it. But we're not. Clearly, we need some help. Help getting started, help getting the most out of every walk, and perhaps most importantly, help creating a walking practice that endures for the rest of our now-potentially-longer-than-they-were-before lives.

How do we get the most out of each walk? Is it better to walk morning, noon, or night? At the mall, on a track, or in the woods? Should you walk in the dead of winter or during the dog days of summer?

Are there ways to up the ante on a walk, and even if you can, should you?

What's the difference between a walk and a hike, and does it matter? Should you strive to become a flâneur or head out to coddiwomple?

Yup, there's a lot to this walking thing.

Mechanics & Form

When my son was about eight months old, my mother-in-law invited us to join her on a cruise. We went. In retrospect, that seems a bit nuts. He was one of those kids who never stopped moving, crawling, and climbing. Never. And here we were aboard a ship where he splashed nonstop in the kiddie pool and crawled at warp speed down the seemingly infinite hallways. Then, seemingly out of the blue, he stood up and started walking. Wobbly at first, but in what seemed like a flash, he was off.

At the time, I couldn't wait for him to cross that milestone and begin walking. *What fun to have an upright human toddling around,* I thought. Hah. Little did I know that once they start walking, the required vigilance escalates dramatically. They transition into the stage that I call "full mobility with zero judgment." It is staggering the danger, trouble, and near misses they manage to stumble into. In retrospect, I have no idea why I was anxious for him to start walking. But he was my first, so I suppose I didn't have a whole lot of judgment either.

Anyway, I remember those first few days. You could practically see the smoke coming out of his ears as his brain worked to figure this walking thing out.

What if I grab this chair leg and pull myself up. Hey, look at that, I'm up. Letting go now. Look at me! Wobbly, but up. Oops, if I lean too far back, I go down on my bum. Okay, let's try that again. Yay! Up again. Oh, wait, if I lean too far forward, I fall on my face. Again, again, again. Ah, here's the balance spot. Crap, I fell over again. Sigh. Now I'm frustrated. But I'm gonna' pull myself up and try again. Got it. Now, can I move this foot forward a bit? One foot, then the other. Hey, look at that! I'm walking!

Once we master walking, it becomes largely automatic, with the many complex elements happening without conscious thought. This alone is remarkable when you consider the many muscles that must work in unison and the constant micro-adjustments that must be made.

Over time, we develop unique walking patterns and habits; some of which serve us, some of which don't. Perhaps our feet turn out a bit, putting additional strain on our ankles and knees. Maybe we angle forward with our gaze on the ground and our shoulders rolled forward. Maybe our quadriceps do all of the work while our hamstrings and glutes confuse walk time with nap time. Maybe we strike the ground flat-footed or tend to walk on the balls of our feet. And then there's our breathing, our arm swing, our gait, our stride ...

So much going on.

Working All the Muscles

When you walk, more than 200 muscles are pressed into service; including your powerful leg muscles: the quadriceps at the front of your thighs, hamstrings at the back of your thighs, glutes at your seat, and the gastrocnemius and soleus in your calves. But those are far, far from all. Also at work are the erector muscles that support your spine and help keep you upright, all five of your primary abdominal muscles, and your often-neglected pelvic floor. The muscles of your shoulders help swing your arms back and forth to maintain the rhythm and balance of your walk while your biceps help you maintain that slightly bent arm position. All of these major muscles are supported by others most of us have never heard of – underappreciated muscles like the psoas, iliacus, and piriformis – plus more than two dozen muscles in our feet and ankles, eight different muscles that support our shoulders, and many, many others.

There is magic in the way all of these muscles and systems work in harmony, with virtually no conscious thought. But understanding the mechanics behind how that magic happens enables us to get the most out of walking and to do it as safely as possible for as long as possible.

To begin to understand the basics, I consulted Sarah Zahab, a Registered Kinesiologist, Clinical Exercise Physiologist, co-founder of Continuum Fitness & Movement Performance, and a nationally-ranked, champion racewalker. Not surprisingly, Sarah has a few thoughts about the mechanics of walking.

Posture: Beach Balls, Balloons, & Breathing

When we talk about posture, we are referring, generally, to our body's alignment, from the top of our heads to the bottom of our feet.

Posture is critical to our long-term wellness, as poor posture, especially over time, can lead to back pain, headaches, poor sleep, deterioration of our spine, compromised balance, and even disruptions to our digestive system. If that's not enough, poor posture can contribute to constipation and incontinence.

Yikes.

"Ideally," Sarah begins, "we should pay attention to our posture throughout our entire day. Improving our walking posture helps us tune in to correct posture and enables us to bring that improved posture into the rest of our lives."

Here's how.

Before you head out on a walk, take a moment to align your body. This is important because, Sarah explains, it is almost impossible to consciously think about firing the correct postural muscles while you walk, so "better alignment at the start helps us to access the right muscles in a more automated and coordinated fashion."

Stack your shoulders over your hips, be sure your chin is parallel to the ground, and imagine a string from the very top of your head putting you tall. Check that you are neither bent over at the waist, pitching your upper body forward, nor arching your back and sticking out your chest or belly. "The goal," Sarah explains, "is to align our ears, shoulders, hips, knees, and ankles and to get those structures stacked on top of one another."

The best way to begin is by focusing on ribs over hips. "When the diaphragm is directly positioned over the pelvic floor," Sarah explains, "your deep intrinsic core muscles can fire optimally."

Once positioned for success, how do we be sure that we engage those core muscles to continue to help us maintain that perfect posture? That's a little tricky – simply sucking in your stomach will not do it. Try this instead: on the count of three, reach your arms out to the side and imagine that you are catching a giant, heavy beach ball that is coming right toward your belly button. One, two, three, catch. If you are like most people, at the moment of imagined impact, your abs will engage. This is a wonderful exercise to do just before you head out on your walk each and every time to remind your abs that they need to get to work.

Okay, abs engaged. But that's not the whole story. Muscles – including our abs and core – are meant to contract and relax. "People, especially women, tend to contract and grip our abs," Sarah explains, "which affects our overall intra-abdominal pressure and can impact other areas such as the pelvic floor (too much downward pressure), the low back (too much backwards pressure), and the abdominal wall (too much forward pressure)."

So, while our abs and core have to be engaged and working, we also need them to relax and expand as we breathe.

Like our beach ball exercise, imagery is helpful here too. "When your lungs fill up with air, imagine two balloons," Sarah explains. "We need expansion, modulation, malleability, and movement on inhalation. The balloons need to open in a 360-fashion, otherwise the pressure gets shifted around and sometimes excess pressure gets placed on other areas."

Ribs over hips.

Abs engaged.

360-degree expansion on every breath.

Check.

Gait

Frankenstein. Charlie Chaplin. Your favorite – or not-so-favorite – clown. Picture them and notice the distinctive and odd way they walk.

"Gait" refers to the overall walking manner or pattern – essentially what happens during the entire cycle of taking steps forward, over and over. Your gait has two phases: the Stance Phase and Swing Phase. The Stance Phase is the moment when the foot is on the ground and it typically comprises about 60% of the walking cycle. The Swing Phase occurs from the time that foot leaves until it once again makes contact with the ground.

Everyone's gait is a little bit different and that is okay. According to Sarah, the most important aspect of gait is that we "land with our center of mass right over our base of support." This helps regulate load and impact, keeps us better aligned, creates a more robust core connection, and allows us to walk more powerfully.

The simplest way to do that? It goes back to posture. When you walk, strive to have your foot land beneath your hips which enables you to maintain the important posture we just talked about and prevent overstriding.

Which leads us to ...

Stride

When I was in college, my boyfriend was 6' 2" – nearly a full foot taller than me. One day, as we were rushing to class, I realized that I took two steps to his every one. Fortunately, I was from New York, while he was from the South, so I tended to walk twice as fast and generally had no difficulty keeping up with him. Our walking speed – our "pace" – is a function of stride and cadence and while his stride was far greater than mine, my pace was faster than his.

Stride is the distance you cover when you take two steps – one with each foot.

Stride is sometimes confused with "step length." Step length is the distance between the point where one foot touches the ground and the next foot touches the ground – essentially the distance you cover with one step. Ideally, your step length should be the same for both sides – you should cross the same distance whether you lead with your right foot or your left.

Both your stride and your step length are functions of several factors including your height, your age, injuries, imbalances, and habit. Many people find that their strides change a bit throughout their walk as they warm up or encounter different terrain.

Being mindful of your stride is important to avoid two relatively common walking errors: overstriding and understriding. Overstriding is more typical, and, according to Sarah, poses the greater risk of injury.

Picture this: you are out for a walk and decide to build in some intervals by adding bursts of faster walking. Well done, as we will explore in a bit, intervals are a terrific way to reap added benefits from your walking practice. In an effort to go faster, you begin to take longer steps:

you increase your stride length so you can cover more distance with fewer steps. This might, at first blush, seem like a good strategy, but it's not. Overstriding disrupts your natural mechanics. It can cause you to strike the ground harder and reduce the natural shock absorption provided by your feet. Over time, this can cause injury to your shins, hips, and back.

Sarah explains that "when we overstride, we often fail to land with our foot beneath our center of mass. This can put more strain on the back and makes it more challenging to recruit the core and hip muscles to do their jobs as stabilizers and prime movers." In other words, it is very difficult to maintain that all-important posture and alignment when we overstride.

How do you know if you are overstriding? As you take a step, your front foot should greet the ground heel first beneath your hip and your knee should remain flexed. If you are stepping so far in front that your heel strikes the ground with force, your front leg lands beyond your body's center of gravity or your knee locks straight, chances are good that you are over-striding.

Sarah suggests experimenting. "Try taking smaller steps and see how you feel overall. Then try much bigger steps and see if you feel a difference in your body. What feels more stable and efficient?"

There are times when you might adjust your gait and stride for changes in conditions or terrain. Last week, I was hiking a mountain trail and as I came down, there was a stretch that was relatively steep with loose rocks and dirt. Realizing that I was at greater risk of slipping, I shortened my stride, widened the space between my feet and kept my knees slightly bent. This gave me better traction and better balance. And I slowed way, way down. When I returned to a flat portion of the trail, I once again focused on stacking shoulders over hips, hips over knees, and gaze forward.

Stride, step length, and gait all adjusted for the terrain. Posture aligned.

Onward.

Feet First

Can we pause for a moment and consider how miraculous our feet are? Seriously, take a moment and look at them. They are tiny as compared to the rest of our bodies, typically between about 9 and 10 inches for women and 10 and 11 inches for men. Despite their diminutive size, those two feet support your entire body weight, often for hours, day in and day out.

By the numbers, our feet have 26 bones, 33 joints, and more than 100 muscles, ligaments, and tendons. They strike the ground with force equivalent to somewhere between four and seven times your body weight and can absorb several *tons* of impact each day.

They could not be more important. And yet, most of us get up every day, shove them into a pair of ill-fitting shoes, and forget about them.

They deserve better.

Let's start with choosing shoes for both walking and for life. Years ago, my high-school daughter decided to take a season off from playing field hockey to run track instead. We spent more than an hour in the local running store trying on shoes. I think she tried on every single pair of size eights they had, before settling on a pair from a top running shoe manufacturer.

"They're perfect," she said, hugging the box to her chest.

Except they weren't. Within a week of daily training, she developed a host of problems, from shin splints to knee problems. She changed shoes and the problems resolved. There was nothing wrong with those shoes per se, but there was a whole lot wrong with those shoes for *her*.

I am often asked, "What are the best shoes for walking?" And my response is always the same: there isn't one because what is best for one person is not necessarily best for someone else.

To learn more about what to look for when choosing a pair of walking shoes, I consulted functional podiatrist and author of *Barefoot Strong*, Dr. Emily Splichal, who explained that "there are a host of factors that go into choosing the right walking shoe, including a person's injury history, foot shape, personal preference, and anticipated walking surface."

"Walking is a repetitive, linear movement," Dr. Splichal explains, so most people benefit from a stiffer, more stable shoe. She suggests looking for a relatively wide toe box (one that doesn't squash your toes), enough cushion to feel comfortable, and a heel counter (the very back of the shoe) that comfortably secures your heel.

And when you find the perfect shoe? Dr. Splichal advises her patients to invest in two pairs and alternate daily because every shoe will be a little bit different and will wear a little bit differently. "By alternating, you may reduce the repetitive impact."

I'm with Dr. Splichal. I alternate between a few different pairs of walking shoes. Of course, I select my walking shoes based on the weather: warmer for winter, cooler for summer, more traction when I know the roads might be slick, older shoes when I know the trails will be muddy. But I also change them up because I want my feet to absorb impact from slightly different angles and at slightly different points of contact.

Once you've laced up those shoes and strolled out the door, begin to notice how your feet greet the ground. You are looking to make initial contact with the heel first. As you move forward, allow your weight to roll through your entire front foot.

Ideally, your feet should remain parallel to one another as you walk, with your toes pointing forward with each step. For many, this will not be the case. Perhaps hips, ankles, knees, or simply habit cause your feet to turn out a bit or turn in a bit. If that is you, it might be worthwhile to visit a podiatrist or orthopedist to help figure out what is going on, as over time those small issues can add up to big problems.

Like any part of your body, your feet can become stronger, more supple, and more flexible with intentional exercise. Yup, exercises for your feet.

There are lots of ideas out there for how to strengthen your feet. You can pretend to draw the alphabet with your big toe, practice picking up marbles with your toes, or simply flex your foot up and down.

According to Dr. Splichal, "Those are fine. But the three most effective exercises I recommend are the Forward Lean, the Short Foot, and the One-Legged Short Foot."

To practice the Forward Lean, begin by standing barefoot with your feet shoulder width apart. Strive to find your "foot tripod" by equally pressuring the base of your big toe, the base of your fifth (little) toe and your heel. Keeping your body stiff as a board, lean forward (imagine the position of a ski-jumper in the air, though not as far forward). "This simple movement activates a postural reflex that activates the muscles of the foot and ankle," Dr. Splichal explains. Repeat three to five times.

To practice the Short Foot exercise, you will once again begin by finding that tripod with the base of your big toe, fifth toe, and heel. Then simply push the tips of your toes down into the ground. You will feel the muscles of your foot turn on and may feel the arch of your foot come up. Hold for 5 seconds, relax and repeat, working up to five times on each foot. Bonus points for contracting your abdominal muscles at the same time as "that helps to integrate our feet (foundation) with our core (center of gravity)," Dr. Splichal explains.

Finally, the One-Legged Short Foot exercise is, well, just like it sounds ... doing the Short Foot exercise standing on one foot. This can be challenging, so place a hand on something for balance, especially as you are beginning to practice these exercises.

If, like most people, you've ignored those 26 bones, 33 joints, and more than 100 muscles, ligaments, and tendons of your feet, start slowly. Don't overstretch those puppies and don't overwork them. But let's stop neglecting them.

Benefits of Barefoot

For as long as I can remember, the beach has been the place where I have found the greatest joy and the greatest peace. I love everything about the ocean: the way the waves are different every day, the squawk of the seagulls, the briny smell, and the way my bare feet feel on the sand. I can walk for hours along the ocean's edge. Apparently, all that barefoot walking is really good for me.

To better understand the benefits of barefoot, I consulted Daniel E. Lieberman, a Professor of Biological Sciences and chair of the Department of Human Evolutionary Biology at Harvard University.

In 2010, Professor Lieberman published a groundbreaking study that examined the impact of running barefoot versus running in cushioned running shoes. His analysis revealed that people tend to strike the ground with more force and in a different way when wearing cushioned sneakers.

Indeed, our ancestors walked and ran for miles without the thickly-padded shoes we've become accustomed to and yet didn't appear to suffer from the types of knee, hip, and back issues that are so common today. How much of that is caused by the shoes we wear versus the sedentary lifestyle we typically live versus something else entirely? It is impossible to know, but there are many who believe that our comfy, cozy, bouncy shoes are not helping us.

I asked Professor Lieberman when we humans began wearing shoes and why. He explained: "Since footwear doesn't preserve well, we don't know for certain, but there is indirect evidence that some form of footwear was present by the origins of the Upper Paleolithic (also known as the Later Stone Age), which starts about 50,000 years ago. Early footwear was probably moccasins or sandals." So early on, we began trying to protect our feet, which seems like a good idea because, despite the fact that our feet can adapt to being barefoot for long stretches, sharp rocks, twigs, and thorns can be hazardous and cause injury.

But walking in shoes does change the way we walk. In a study that sought to investigate the impact of walking in shoes versus walking barefoot on our Achilles tendon (the tendon that runs up the back of our ankles), researchers discovered that walking with shoes "resulted in significant changes in several basic gait parameters" including lower cadence, greater stride and step length, 12% longer step duration, and increased ankle flexion as compared to walking barefoot. The researchers concluded that typical running shoes increased the load on the Achilles tendon.

It appears that walking barefoot can deliver a host of other benefits as well.

Walking barefoot can strengthen the many muscles of the feet, keeping them strong and flexible.

Walking barefoot can also improve balance, both as a result of those stronger and more responsive muscles and because bare feet provide a better sense of where our body is in space and improve our ability to sense movement, a concept known as proprioception.

Walking barefoot also helps to strengthen the muscles of our legs – especially our lower legs.

Walking barefoot can improve the mechanics of our walking, encouraging us to greet the ground in a more natural way and roll forward through the front of our feet. This can decrease impact and may decrease our potential for injury.

Finally, there is an emerging body of research that suggests walking barefoot on natural surfaces, like grass, soil, or the beach – sometimes called "earthing" or "grounding" – offers a host of health and wellness benefits including reduced inflammation, improved immune responses, accelerated wound healing, better sleep, increased energy, and improved blood chemistry. How? Researchers aren't entirely sure, but the working hypothesis is that grounding enables our bodies to absorb ions from the earth that results in a myriad of positive physical impacts.

But don't throw out your favorite walking shoes and take to the trails just yet. As Professor Lieberman explains, "Like everything, being barefoot or shod has both costs and benefits. The biggest benefit of being barefoot is increased sensory perception. But the cost is less protection and (usually) comfort." Especially if you've been walking in thickly-padded shoes, transitioning to safely walking barefoot is going to take time. "If you decide to increase how much you walk barefoot, be sure to do so slowly and gradually," Professor Lieberman advises. Avoid places with sharp rocks and broken glass and build slowly to give your body plenty of time to adjust to new walking mechanics and your feet time to build the strength and calluses needed for protection.

How Far, How Fast, How Often?

How often should I walk? How far do I have to go to start to feel better and live longer? What do I have to do to lose weight by walking? How fast should I walk? How many miles should I walk each day? Each week? Each month? Each year? And remind me again about that 10,000 steps a day thing?

I get these questions a lot. And by a lot, I mean practically every day.

Every Walk "Makes a Difference"

Recently, I was interviewed by a national women's magazine about walking. The writer asked why walking is a great form of exercise. I shared the many benefits of walking for your mind, mood, and body and we chatted about the many muscles we use when we walk, and why I'm a proponent of an intentional walking practice.

Then she asked, "How long does it take to make a difference?"

This question stumped me. "Every walk makes a difference," I replied after a pause. "Every walk fires up your happiness hormones, reduces your cortisol, improves your mood, gives you the chance to be present and clear your mind, boosts your creativity, engages dozens and dozens of muscles, reduces your blood sugar, works your heart ... I could go on and on," I said.

"But summer is coming, so how much walking does it take to really, you know, make a difference?"

That was when I realized what she was actually getting at. The question she really wanted to ask was more along the lines of, "How many walks does it take to lose weight or make a noticeable *visible* difference?" Sigh.

When are we going to stop measuring the value of moving our bodies based on how that movement makes us *look* and begin valuing movement based on how it makes us *feel*?

Over the past decade or so, countless articles and experts have been espousing the importance of self-care. We are being reminded that you "can't pour from an empty cup," that you have to "put your mask on first before taking care of others" and a host of other platitudes about the importance of self-care. I have spoken, written, lectured, and cajoled on these very same points. This is important work. For decades before, people – and women in particular – have been told that in order to be a good wife, mother, daughter, friend, employee, manager, entrepreneur, we need to put ourselves last. It is high time for that narrative to change.

When we talk about the importance of self-care, we tend to focus on things like saying no, giving ourselves time for a bubble bath or a good book, putting ourselves first, at least from time to time. All of these things are important. Self-care is critical to your well-being and however self-care looks for you is great.

Yet when we talk about moving our bodies – about physical activity – our focus shifts to how long will it take to lose weight and *look* better?

This is how we've been conditioned away from appreciating the joy that comes from a walk. We've been indoctrinated into a culture that focuses on movement to serve our outward self and have lost the connection to how movement makes us feel. Viewing the power of physical activity through that lens, when we don't immediately see visible changes, we convince ourselves that our walking practice isn't "making a difference."

We must stop asking ourselves "How often do I need to walk to look better in a bathing suit?" Instead, we need to start asking ourselves,

"How much better do I feel when I walk?" We have to rediscover how to listen to our bodies. Neither one walk nor a dozen walks will make you look better in a bathing suit. But a lifetime of walking as a practice, a lifetime of better managing your stress, a lifetime of, yes, burning calories every day, a lifetime of bettering your brain will change, extend, and improve your life.

So the actual, true answer to "How much do I need to walk to make a difference?" is this: every single walk makes a difference. Every single one.

That Said ...

Remember the thing about the 10,000 steps a day being an artificial target thought up by a Japanese marketing team? Well, it turns out that they weren't that far off. Over the past few decades, researchers have sought to identify the Holy Grail of daily steps: exactly how many steps should a person take each day to minimize their risk of illness and maximize their lifespan and healthspan?

While there is no one single number of steps that is the magic bullet for all people of all ages to prevent all diseases, studies reveal some guidelines.

Let's begin with the power of small increases for those who have been largely sedentary. For them, dramatic improvements in health and longevity have been observed from moderate increases in their number of daily steps. For instance, in a study that included close to 17,000 older women, those who averaged 4,400 steps per day had "significantly lower mortality rates" than those who averaged 2,700 steps per day. Moreover, as "more steps per day were accrued, mortality rates progressively decreased before leveling at approximately 7,500 steps." This is an important place to begin our discussion because I fear too many people have absorbed the message that if they can't get to 10,000 steps a day, they shouldn't even bother. But they should: every step counts.

For the sake of "all-cause mortality" – a term used in medical research to mean death from any cause – the optimal number of daily steps seems to be somewhere between 6,000 and 9,000 with the exact number being dependent upon age and other factors. Generally, for adults over 60, the reduction in risk appears to level off between 6,000 and 8,000 steps per day, while for those under 60, the reduction in risk plateaus between 8,000 and 10,000 steps.

Another study suggests that 8,200 steps per day is the key threshold associated with the reduced risk of a variety of specific ailments and chronic diseases including obesity, sleep apnea, gastroesophageal reflux disease, major depressive disorder, diabetes, and hypertension, with most – but not all – disease risk continuing to decline as daily-step count increased. Finally, Harvard Medical School interpreted the research to teach us that for people ages 40 and older, "the more steps people took, the lower their risk of dying over the following 10 years, regardless of their age, sex, or race. In fact, compared with people who walked 4,000 steps per day, those who walked 8,000 steps daily were about half as likely to die for any reason – but especially from heart disease."

So, if you really, really want a number, 8,200 daily steps seems to be a pretty good target.

That said, most studies suggest that more steps are better and, as we will explore shortly, intensity matters: you get different benefits when you walk with "moderate intensity" (around 100 steps per minute) or "vigorous intensity" (closer to 130 steps per minute) as compared to when you stroll along letting Rover stop to sniff every bush and pee on every fire hydrant. Intensity of your walk can be increased in other ways that we will explore including adding intervals, hills, stairs, load, or walking poles.

All of this research has focused on the association between total daily-step counts and preventable illness and longevity. Hit the goal on your watch or phone, park at the far end of the parking lot, get in those extra steps.

But.

For the sake of your mental clarity, your overall happiness and all of the other benefits of the intentional walking practice don't just count those steps. Take those intentional walks.

Focus on Frequency, Duration, and Intensity. Or Don't.

Unless you've decided to take up competitive racewalking (which has been an Olympic sport since 1904), you do not have to turn your walking practice into something you constantly measure and strive to "level up." You can be an opportunistic walker who walks out the door whenever the mood strikes (as long as the mood strikes more often than not). You can create a neighborhood walking group. You can walk with your friends and you can walk by yourself. Like creativity researcher and best-selling author Tina Seelig told me, you can "walk when you need to think" or, like Claudia Beeney, you can walk when you need to untangle your thoughts and generate fresh ideas. You can walk when you feel stress and tension rising, or you can walk at the end of the day as a way to transition between work and home. You can take a 10-minute walk after dinner, walk while you catch up by phone with your college roommate, challenge yourself with a long walk in the woods, or join a local hiking club.

Walking is powerful and can impact you in a myriad of positive ways however and whenever you do it. But, as with most forms of exercise, if you want to get a bit more technical and evaluate your walking practice with respect to *physical benefits*, there are three general elements to consider:

- *Frequency* – how often do you walk?
- *Duration* – how long do you walk?
- *Intensity* – how hard do you work when you walk?

Each of these metrics provides a measurable dial you can adjust up or down to develop the walking practice that is best for you.

Frequency: How Often Should You Walk?

As with most things, it depends. Let's start with why you are walking. For your heart health? For your mood? To help regulate your blood sugar or manage your weight? To focus your mind and boost your energy for a crucial afternoon meeting? Walking should be a tool in your personal and professional arsenal that you deploy when you need it. But if we are talking strictly about the health benefits, research does provide some guidelines.

Over the past several decades, researchers have sought to identify exactly how much exercise people should get each week. The most often cited recommendation is that of the U.S. Department of Health and Human Services, which recommends that adults get at least 150 minutes of moderate-intensity aerobic activity, such as walking, and that they spread those 150 minutes out over several sessions, typically 30 minutes each, five times a week. There is much debate over this recommendation, with many experts arguing that this is the bare minimum and that true health and wellness requires far more time invested. Meanwhile, others argue that encouraging people to move their bodies for at least 30 minutes at least three days a week can deliver meaningful benefits over a sedentary lifestyle.

That said, there is a whole lotta' research out there showing that, generally speaking, more is better.

There's a caveat to this: rest and recovery are critical and repeating the same activity, in the same way, day in and day out can lead to repetitive use injuries. Thus, while moving your body most days is ideal, building up to that slowly and changing what you do, how you do it, and where you do it, can be beneficial.

Moreover, as we will discuss, many of us need to consciously reject the all-or-nothing mentality that can impede both our progress and our happiness. For many, setting a goal of walking each and every day, come rain or shine, injury or work deadline, illness or sprained ankle, may derail your intentions and set you up for failure.

So, let's stick with, whenever possible, walking most days is best.

Duration: How Long Should You Walk?

I think we've established that all walking is good walking and the answer to how long you should walk depends on countless factors ranging from your personal level of fitness to how much time you have available. That said, there are benefits to shorter walks and benefits to longer walks.

Benefits of a 10-Minute Walk

We have been told, over and over and again, that physical activity only counts at a certain time and intensity. Many of us have come to believe that if we don't have 30 minutes to get our sweat on, "why bother?" It is simply not true: every minute matters, every walk counts, and all of those steps add up. In fact, there's actually a name for it: "fractionalized exercise." And the evidence continues to mount that tremendous benefits come from even a single 10-minute walk. Manage a few 10-minute walks during the course of the day? Even better.

In fact, at least one study showed that three bouts of 10-minute walking was actually more beneficial for lowering blood pressure than a single 30-minute session. Moreover, according to the Anxiety and Depression Association of America, "Psychologists studying how exercise relieves anxiety and depression suggest that a 10-minute walk may be just as good as a 45-minute workout."

For the more than 30 million Americans with Type 2 diabetes, a study showed that three 10-minute walks following meals lowered blood sugar levels an average of 12% more than a single 30-minute walk each day, with the biggest benefit from a 10-minute after-dinner walk. What about those who don't have diabetes? Does a post-meal short walk help them too? It looks like it does, with at least one study showing that even a short, light intensity walk can materially improve blood sugar levels.

What if we all added a 10 minute walk to our days? A study that analyzed an extensive body of research revealed a starting insight: more than 111,000 deaths would be prevented each year if most Americans added just 10 minutes of physical activity to their days.

Those short walks might be easier to fit into your routine. You don't have to change into some special walking outfit (though good footwear is still important), don't have to get your sweat on, and probably won't need a shower when you're done.

What happens if we truly accept that a 10-minute walk is enough to "make a difference"? What if we begin asking ourselves "what can I do" rather than telling ourselves that we don't have 30 minutes, so "why bother?"

How Long I Typically Walk … and Why

Most days, when I first head out for a walk, my mind bounces all over. I think about the work undone, the dinner unprepared, and the emails unanswered. In winter, I worry that I'm not dressed warmly enough, in summer I contemplate whether or not I remembered to sunblock my ears. Somehow, I manage to feel bored instantly and wish I was sitting in front of my computer working or laying on my couch reading. I consider turning back, but I keep going, reminding myself that I will feel better when the walk is done.

And I practically walk for a living.

Somewhere around the 10-minute mark, I begin to settle in. My mind begins to clear and I relax into the rhythm of the walk. If I tune in closely to my body, I can feel the stress leaving and the positive feelings bubbling up. After about 20 minutes, the ideas begin to flow. By the time I return home, 30 or 40 minutes later, my mind, mood, and body have shifted.

And Then There are the Long Walks

There were ten of us who had come together as strangers just 48 hours earlier. It was day three of a guided hiking trip and today we were tackling eleven dusty miles in a remote area of Canyonlands National Park. Now, I walk regularly, usually four or five days each week, typically between two and three miles. But eleven miles? Up and down mountain trails, through slot canyons, across sweeping desert fields, and scrambling over boulders? Yeah, that sounded like a lot.

The group eyed each other nervously. Though we were mostly silent, I suspect most were thinking the same things I was: Do I have enough water? What about snacks? Am I dressed right? Will I be too hot or too cold? And, most importantly, will I make it?

"Alright," our hiking guide said after a few moments. "Let's go."

History is replete with stories of the long walk. From the pilgrimages of many of the world's religions to Cheryl Strayed's wildly popular memoir *Wild*, the power of a long walk to effectuate personal transformation is as old as recorded history.

Why? How?

First, during a long walk, you have access to all of the brain benefits we explored earlier, your cortisol is lower, your executive function is higher, and you are in the best possible mental space to sort through whatever thoughts, issues, or challenges you need to sort through.

We started out as a group, with a 20-minute gentle climb over immense slabs of rock. Bit by bit, we began to separate as people fell into their own rhythms and conversations began to bubble up in smaller groups. I found myself just in front of a group of three, talking loudly and non-stop. I felt a pull in two directions: slow down and join their conversation, or speed up and take the time to get lost in my own head. I choose the latter, summoning some energy (which I was afraid I might need later) and moving quickly away from the chatty trio. I was craving silence, looking for the chance to allow my mind to clear and find answers, though at that moment, I didn't even know the questions I was looking to answer.

A long walk gives you time and space that we often don't have in our overstuffed days, where our attention is constantly being diverted by this notification or that text. We need more time to think than our modern lives provide. Long stretches of time that enable our minds to wander and our hearts to wonder.

Then there is the physical metaphor that a long walk provides: putting one foot in front of the other and moving forward – literally and figuratively – one step at a time. When we feel unfulfilled and unsatisfied and restless, we say that we feel "stuck." That long walk? Well, there's nothing stuck about it.

Just over an hour into our hike, we began to descend, which is a weird feeling in the middle of a hike. Typically, you go up up up, reach a peak, and then begin the descent. This was different. We picked our way down, grabbing branches for stability, until we found ourselves on a sandy floor where we took a hard left turn into a slot canyon. Rock walls stretched up on either side, blocking out the sun and its warmth. It was like being in a long, narrow hallway.

I am a bit claustrophobic and part of me didn't like it at all. But the other part of me was absorbed by the majesty of the rocks, the colors of the stone, the incongruity of the sandy floor. One foot in front of the other. There were moments when the walls seemed to close in, and others where the sun managed to find an angle through the slots, illuminating the way forward.

How long was I walking through that dimly lit slot canyon? Five minutes? Ten? Thirty? I have no idea, but at some point, I stepped out of the narrow darkness out into the bright sunshine of an enormous open field that stretched as far as I could see in every direction, littered with boulders that looked like sculptures and flowers that seemed impossible in the scorched earth.

Talk about a metaphor.

Intensity: How Hard Should You Work When You Walk?

Yesterday, I took Moose for two separate daily walks.

Walk #1: I dropped my daughter at school at 7:50 and Moose and I went straight to our favorite wooded trail. He was off leash and after just a few minutes of warming up at a slow pace, we picked up the speed to my typical "fitness" walking pace – about three miles per hour. Since we do this walk often, Moose knew the drill and, though he stopped occasionally to sniff, he knew his job was to keep up with me. After about 10 minutes, I noticed that my heart rate was elevated, my breathing was quicker, and my body was warming up. I unzipped my jacket and stuffed my gloves in my pockets. 45 minutes later, we hopped back in the car. This was a walk designed to get my blood pumping, spur my energy and my happiness hormones, and get my mind, mood, and body ready for the day.

Walk #2: After dinner was eaten and dishes were done, Eric and I leashed Moose for an after-dinner stroll. We walked down the dead-end street in front of our house and back – exactly one mile. When Moose stopped to sniff – which he did often – we stopped with him. Chatting the entire way, Eric and I caught up about the day just past and planned the day to come. I have no idea how fast we were moving, but I do know that my breathing never became labored and my voice never became breathy. Gloves stayed on, as did the hat I had pulled down to cover my ears.

Two different walks, two very different levels of intensity.

Intensity refers to how hard your body is working when you are walking (or doing any kind of physical activity) and presents the opportunity for tremendous variation. There is a big difference in intensity between a stroll down the street with Moose as he stops to sniff every leaf, mailbox, and spring flower and my three-mile fitness walk in the woods. Or the difference between an afternoon window-shopping on Main Street and a hike up the side of a mountain.

In walking, intensity is generally a function of two primary things: speed and terrain. Obviously, the more quickly you walk, the harder you are asking your body to work. Just as obvious, walking uphill is more strenuous than walking on a flat surface. Other factors can impact intensity including any load you carry, the surface on which you walk and even the weather: your body typically works harder in the cold or extreme heat than in more moderate temperatures. Finally, intensity is individual, based on your personal level of fitness.

So how much intensity is best?

Once again, it depends. And once again, more is better ... to a point.

Many articles and experts will offer up specific steps per minute as a measure of intensity. This doesn't make much sense because, as we have discussed, intensity is personal and depends on a host of factors beyond simply speed. So if we can't just measure our steps per minute to figure out how hard we are working, what *should* we measure?

Assuming we are talking about the physical benefits of walking – rather than all of the holistic benefits – it is useful to consider walking in the context of "Zone 2 training" which is the phrase that exercise physiologists use to describe sustained physical activity during which you maintain a heart rate between 60 and 70 percent of your maximum. Ascertaining these numbers is based on your personal history, fitness level, and any illnesses or diseases. That said, to estimate your maximum heart rate – assuming you have no confounding conditions – simply subtract your age from 220. Based on this, my maximum target heart rate would be 162.

Next, to figure out my target heart rate for Zone 2 training, I simply calculate 65% of 162. So my Zone 2 training target heart rate is about 105. Obviously, these numbers are general benchmarks: the target Zone 2 heart rate for a 58-year-old marathoner is going to be very different from mine, as will the target Zone 2 heart rate for a 58-year-old who is just beginning her fitness journey after years at a sedentary job.

While I know there is value in ascertaining just how hard my heart is working, I hate to fire up a heart-rate monitor and check it during my walk because doing so interferes with my ability to be fully present and able to reap all of the other benefits that walk offers. Fortunately, the so-called "Talk Test" provides a far easier, yet surprisingly reliable, measure of exertion.

If your body is working at "low-intensity" you will be able to speak in full sentences without sounding breathy or needing to pause for breath.

If your body is working at "moderate-intensity," à la Zone 2, you will be able to maintain a conversation, but you will sound "breathy" and may need to pause speaking from time to time to catch your breath.

If your body is working at "high-intensity," words come out only one or two at a time between breaths and you are unable to maintain a conversation.

I know, sounds simple right?

While all walking "counts" and all walking is beneficial, if we are looking to maximize the benefits of our walking practice, especially for our bodies, intensity does matter. And there are several ways to increase that intensity and get a little bit more bang for your walking buck.

Up the Ante

Last spring, I was in New Orleans, visiting my dearest childhood friend, Lorelei. The people of New Orleans – at least in my experience – take their leisure and their fun far more seriously than the people of New York do. The Tuesday morning of our visit, Lorelei announced that she had made reservations at one of her favorite restaurants. "I reserved the table on the porch," she said, "and invited a few friends." There were nine people in total: my family, including our 16-year-old daughter, Lorelei's family, and a few friends. The meal lasted more than two hours. On a Tuesday. I loved it.

Nevertheless, old habits die hard and my desire to accomplish as much as possible in as short a time as possible persists. So sure, I walk for my mental and emotional health, but I can't help asking myself ... How can I get more bang for my walking buck? Are there ways to increase the physical intensity of my walks, convert them into full-body workouts, and heighten their heart-strengthening, bone-building impact?

There are.

Incline: Adding incline to a walk is an incredibly effective way to increase the physical challenge – you'll get stronger and you'll burn more calories. So along your walk, if you see a set of stairs, take them. If you see a hill, climb it.

Intervals: Changing up the speed at various points during your walk is another effective way to increase the challenge. Interval training has been shown to help your cardiovascular system grow even stronger, teach your body to recover more quickly, and burn more calories.

A Weighted Pack: Adding a weighted backpack – especially one specifically designed to be worn while walking – is a tremendously effective way to increase the intensity of your walk and to activate additional back, core, and shoulder muscles. Often called "rucking," it has been a staple of military physical fitness training for millenia. Start with a light weight and increase both the weight and distance slowly over time.

Walking Poles: Here's the walking pole paradox: walking poles make your walk seem easier, while at the same time engaging many, many more muscles and significantly increasing the caloric burn.

What about adding hand or ankle weights? Most experts don't rec-ommend it unless you keep those weights quite light, no more than a pound or two at the most. While ankle or hand weights can increase the intensity of your walk – you are moving more weight through space – the research suggests that adding more than a couple of pounds can put additional, unnecessary strain on your joints – most notably your ankles, knees, elbows, neck, and shoulders. Weights can also throw off your natural walking gait and, over time, the repetitive motion and ad-ditional strain can negatively impact your back, hips, and shoulders. In short, the slight benefit you might get is probably not worth the risk to your very precious joints.

When To Walk?

Morning, Noon, or Night

The short answer is you should walk whenever is most convenient for you. Build whatever routine, practice, or habit you can sustain. If that means you get up in the morning, pull on your walking gear before you have the chance to talk yourself out of it and head immediately out the door, great. If you walk after work as a way to stretch and strengthen muscles that have been sitting too long or shake off the stress of the day, fantastic. If you walk after dinner with a loved one as a way to connect, that's good too.

Like I said, pretty much all walking is good walking.

Yet there are some unique benefits to walking at different times of the day. Let's explore.

Rise & Shine: The Benefits of Walking in the Morning

I am a morning person. I love the peace and quiet of predawn when the rest of my house and much of the world around me is still sleeping. My mind is clear, the coffee is hot, and I am often my happiest and most clear-headed. On the best days, after an hour or two of work and writing, I will lace up my sneakers and head out into the morning light for a two-mile walk. Not always, but when I manage that routine, I find I am my most productive, most creative, and most cheerful throughout the day. Coincidence? I don't think so.

I'm not alone. In a recent survey of more than 300 women who maintain a regular walking practice, 68% of them prefer a morning walk, including Lynda Brady whose early morning walks "set the tone for the day. I reflect on my life, talk with God, and plan. If I don't walk by 7 a.m., my entire day is off."

Regular walker Dominique Butts describes her early morning walking practice in this way: "There's a hushed serenity to the early morning that I find rejuvenating, reflective, and peaceful. Listening to the birds herald in the sunrise and watching the sky gradually illuminate makes me feel that I can accomplish anything! This mindset fuels my ability to remain open, mindful, and connected throughout the day."

Others like Tany Wine crave the ease and solitary nature of an early morning walk. She explains that, "I walk early in the morning, before work. I'm out the door a little before 6, home before 7, and showered and at work by 7:30. I walk on residential streets and I like that in the early hours, they are mostly empty. Since I don't expect to see anyone, I basically roll out of bed, get dressed, and get out the door. I don't wash my face or brush my teeth. I'm not putting on my 'game face' and there's nothing else competing for my attention. Walking first thing gives me a sense of accomplishment right out the gate and when I finish, I feel awake and energized. No matter what else happens that day, good or bad, at least I got my walk in."

Lynda, Dominique, and Tany and the millions of other early morning walkers are onto something.

First, those who walk, or who engage in any type of intentional physical activity first thing in the morning, are more likely to stick with it. Why? Probably because you get your exercise in before the demands of the day interfere – and there will always be demands of the day.

Second, an early morning walk can also help to set your circadian rhythm, which can boost your energy during the day and help you sleep better at night. As explained in a 2008 paper on the benefits of sunlight, "We humans are programmed to be outdoors while the sun is shining and home in bed at night." Exposure to daylight halts our body's production of melatonin, the hormone that helps tell us when it is time to be asleep and when it is time to be awake. "When people are exposed to sunlight … in the morning, their nocturnal melatonin production occurs sooner, and they enter into sleep more easily at night," which helps people fall asleep sooner and sleep better. Setting your circadian rhythm with exposure to morning sunlight has been shown to be effective against insomnia, premenstrual syndrome, and seasonal affective disorder.

Then there are the practical considerations. In hot climates – especially in the summer months – the early morning walks often offer the best chance to beat the heat and, if you live in a relatively urban environment, pollution levels tend to be at their lowest first thing in the morning.

For many people, early morning walks are easier to fit into their lives and to maintain, as they will often be out the door before the whirlwind of the day has the chance to disrupt their plans. That is certainly true for Tany who explains that, "In the evening after work, other house-hold chores and time with family compete for my time. But not at 6 in the morning."

Ladies Who Lunch ... Walk

If you sat down at your desk at 9:00, by mid-day, you have likely used a whole lot of mental energy. Not to mention, if your job is fairly sedentary, you've been sitting for three hours or more. Physically and mentally, it is time for a break and a lunchtime walk can be precisely what you need to spark your creativity, boost your energy and improve your decision making – a perfect mid-day prescription. It works for Shannon Riggs who cherishes her lunchtime walks. "Taking a break in the middle of the workday to get outside feels like a treat. It allows me to stretch after sitting at my desk, and helps me focus better during the second half of the day."

Even if your work has you on your feet, that mid-day walk can boost your energy and provide the mental and emotional break you need. It certainly did for a group of nurses at a mid-Western hospital.

I interviewed one who shared this story. "Years ago, a group of nurses started a mid-day walking group. Every day, we meet and walk and talk. It's been great for all of us. We connect and feel like we have support, and get to walk off some of the stress from the day. Most of us have even lost a little bit of weight. And over time, we've become good friends. Honestly, those walks have changed our work-life." I asked her what they do on the days when the weather makes it impossible to walk outside. Laughing, she said, "We discovered a loop in the basement and we walk there. It's not nearly as nice as being outside, but it is much better than not going." Where there's a will, there's a way.

Depending on where you live and the time of year, mid-day can offer the best walking weather, especially in colder months and climates.

What about those whose work requires clothing and make up that might not be the ideal for a vigorous walk? Is it worth going out for a moderate 15-minute walk that doesn't get your sweat on? Absolutely: even a leisurely 15-minute mid-day walk is going to deliver improved energy, focus, and concentration for the afternoon.

Happy Hour: Benefits of a Late Afternoon Walk

Sometimes the text goes out earlier in the day, but typically it is closer to 3:30 or 4:00. "Wanna' walk – 4:30 Barcelona?" Often, I'm the one to send it to one of my usual walking partners. It's an act of will because, by the time 3:15 rolls around, the last thing I feel like doing is going for a walk. At that time of day, I feel simultaneously that I still have tons of work left to do in the office and dinner to plan at home. And 3:30 puts me squarely in the midst of the mid-afternoon slump.

The mid-afternoon slump is a real thing, caused by a combination of a circadian rhythm telling you it is time to start winding down, a brain that has become fatigued by a day of work and decision making, and a body that has had a day's worth of cortisol coursing through it. Many people experience fatigue, impaired focus, poor decision-making, increased stress, or mood disruption and often crave a quick fix – sugar and caffeine being the most common.

Everyone is different and there are those who don't experience an energy crash, but rather find their energy, focus, and productivity peak during the late afternoon. But those people are the exception: Most of us experience the mid-afternoon slump that sends us running for a cookie, a cup of coffee, or a nap.

A walk can be more effective. As we have already mentioned, one study compared 10-minutes of stair walking to the caffeine equivalent of a shot of espresso. Walking won. Walking also helps improve executive function, reduce stress hormones, increase positive hormones, restore your decision-making capacity, and boost your creativity, making it much, much easier to answer the age-old question, "What's for dinner?"

So no, as 3:30 rolls around, the last thing I typically feel like doing is lacing up my sneakers and heading out for a walk. That is why a walk with friends is perfect for this time of day, 'cause if I'm not committed to someone else, chances are good that a cookie will win over the better boost that comes from a walk.

A happy-hour walk also provides a potent way to transition from work to home. It gives you the chance to process the day. Especially for those with stressful jobs, a post-work, pre-dinner walk offers the chance to leave that stress on the trail and fire up their happiness hormones before they walk in the door.

It works for Dawniel Baker who strives to find an hour to walk no matter what time she gets done with work so she can "fully transition to home with a clear head and a happy heart."

Donna Norton agrees. "Walking right after work clears my mind and creates a nice separation between work and the rest of my day."

For many, the trick to making that post-work walk happen is to keep the momentum of the day going. Teacher Jan Grey explains, "I just change shoes and keep work clothes on. If I sit down too long, I won't go back out." Jaime Butts agrees. "I take clothes and change so I can walk right after work. If I get all the way home, chances are that I won't leave the house again."

Grandma Was Right: The Benefits of an After-Dinner Walk

In our house, most evenings go like this: Dinner is eaten, dishes are washed, the kitchen is cleaned, coffee is set up to brew in the morning, and I head straight to bed with a book or a television show.

This is not ideal. Not at all ideal.

Better would be taking the advice of my grandmother and heading out for an after-dinner walk because, though she certainly didn't have the science to understand it, her instincts were right: an after-dinner walk can have profound, positive impact on our minds, moods, and bodies.

First, after-dinner walks taken with family members provide a perfect time to catch up and connect. As we will discover, walking together is valuable for relationships and, while it doesn't matter when you walk together, after dinner presents an opportune time for many. For young kids, an evening walk can help create a lifelong habit. For teenagers, an after-dinner walk can help them power through evening homework.

Second, an after-dinner walk can help promote digestion by helping to keep things moving through your digestive tract. Research suggests that a post-meal walk helps to speed up the emptying of your stomach and can reduce bloating. This is not the case with everyone, nor with every meal – whether an after-dinner walk feels good or bad can depend on how much you've eaten and how your unique body processes food. Once you develop the after-dinner walk routine, you will begin to recognize what meals walk well and what meals don't. Chances are that you'll discover that meals that are higher in vegetables, lean proteins, and good grains walk a whole lot better than a plate of fried chicken, mashed potatoes, and gravy.

Finally, and perhaps most importantly for your body, is the impact that a walk following a meal can have on your blood sugar levels. After a meal, your blood sugar levels typically rise, as your body gets to work converting food to energy. This is a normal bodily function, however larger blood sugar spikes can contribute to cardiovascular disease, diabetes, and other not-so-good for your diseases and disorders. Helping our bodies better process the food we take in and keep those blood sugar levels steadier helps to avoid these diseases and disorders. Several studies have shown that a post-meal walk of merely 15 or 20 minutes helps.

Yup, once again, Grandma was right.

And Then There are the Night Owls

Walking late in the evening presents challenges with weather, darkness, and safety. Nevertheless, for people like Julie Stecher, late night walks offer the best respite from her hectic life. She explains, "I like to take my walk at night. I go at 10 pm. I have a full-time job by day, and take care of my mother during my off time. Life can be hectic and stressful. I have found that walking at this time not only relieves the stress, but also relaxes me and helps me sleep."

There are few things as calm and peaceful as a late night walk. The world of humans is quiet and the sounds of nature are loud. The world appears different than it does during our hectic days. You can appreciate the stars, observe the moon in its different phases, and perhaps even catch the occasional shooting star. You can appreciate that you are both small in the vastness of the universe, yet somehow connected – the perfect recipe to experience awe.

Late night walking is not without its potential for hazards. Be cautious and be smart. Stick to well-lit areas, stay alert to your surroundings, and always suit up with lights or reflective gear that faces both front and back.

Walking Winter, Spring, Summer, or Fall

She was very particular. She didn't like her porridge too hot or too cold, her chair too big or too small, or her bed too hard or too soft. I suspect if she had a regular walking practice, Goldilocks wouldn't walk if it was too hot or too cold, too wet or too snowy, too dark or too windy.

Don't be like Goldilocks. While there are certainly days when Mother Nature says heck no to walking – frigid temperatures with windchill making it worse, sleet, wind strong enough to take down branches, black ice coating roads and sidewalks, heat that sears your shoulders within moments, rain accompanied by thunder and lightning – most days, the right clothes, gear, and attitude are all you need.

Winter Walking: Why You Should You Walk in the Cold

When it is cold, millions of years of evolution compels us to seek shelter and stay cozy in the cave. Our operating system tries to insist that we move as little as possible, don't expend unnecessary energy, and eat up because who knows when and where our next meal is coming. We need to fight that urge. We need to push ourselves to remain active because – beyond all of the things we've already talked about – walking in cold weather has even more benefits. Here are six.

Many of Us Need the Mood Boost

According to the American Psychiatric Association, about 5% of Americans suffer from Seasonal Affective Disorder and experience symptoms similar to those of depression during the short, dark days of winter. Many, many others experience milder winter blues. While experts don't fully understand the exact mechanism that causes the winter blues or full-blown Seasonal Affective Disorder, they believe it is connected to the reduced exposure to daylight, which can disrupt our bodies' natural rhythms and impact the hormones that affect our sleep and our mood. What they do know is that exercise and exposure to sunlight can both help. Walking outside delivers both.

Bring on the Vitamin D

Vitamin D is crucial for good health, and since it's not an easy vitamin to get through your diet, sun exposure is key. Research shows that just ten to thirty minutes of sunlight several times each week can help you get the Vitamin D you need – with exactly how much depending on how sensitive your skin is. Sunlight through a window doesn't trigger Vitamin D production. A daily walk outside does.

Increase the Calorie Burn

Walking does so much more than burn calories, but balancing our calorie intake with our calorie outtake is essential to maintaining a healthy weight. Walking can help, and perhaps even more so in the winter. Because your body is also working to stay warm, research suggests that a cold weather walk burns more calories.

Activate Your Immune System

As we discussed earlier, walking has been shown to strengthen your immune system and reduce inflammation – a great combination when winter increases our exposure to cold germs. But we might receive an added boost from walking in the cold. How? Turns out that regular exposure to cold can have a positive impact on our immune system.

Exactly how effective walking in the cold may be is yet to be determined but, in this context, it appears our mothers may have been wrong: going out in the cold might not cause you to catch your death of cold, but to the contrary, it might help you combat that cold.

The Benefits of Brown

Not that many years ago, researchers identified brown adipose tissue, otherwise known as brown fat. While the research is nascent, initial research suggests that this type of fat tissue helps our bodies regulate heat and may play a role in how our bodies use and store energy, with more brown fat enabling us to better metabolize glucose and, perhaps, help us to maintain a healthy weight. At the very least, initial studies indicate that more brown fat is good for us. One of the things that can help us create more brown fat? Exposure to cold.

See a Different World

"Let's go snowshoeing," Tom suggested. We were guests at his family's lodge in the Adirondack mountains of upstate New York. It was January, so it was cold and there were places where the snow drifts were waist deep.

We bundled up in ski pants and parkas, strapped old-fashioned snow-shoes to our boots, and walked out the front door. Halfway down the long driveway, we took a left onto a snow-covered trail and into a magical winter wonderland. Seriously, Disney had nothing on this view. The trees looked like sculptures hung with infinite diamonds that sparkled in the sun and the quiet was preternatural. It was some of Mother Nature's most spectacular work that you will only discover if you fight the urge to stay safe and warm in your cave.

But Do Consider This

There are critical safety concerns to consider before you venture out in the cold.

Most importantly, doing any kind of physical activity in the cold places additional strain on your heart and respiratory systems, so if you are compromised in any way, check with your doctor before heading out for cold weather walking. Build up to winter-time walking slowly. Maintaining your walking practice through the fall as the temperature drops bit by bit helps.

And when you do venture out in the winter cold remember:

- **Beware the Ice.** Winter walking can be treacherous. Watch out for ice, especially "black ice" on roads that can be difficult to see. Assume that anything that looks wet or shiny is likely icy and avoid it if possible. If your path requires you to traverse an icy patch, take smaller steps, keep your knees slightly bent, and slow down your pace. Keep your hands out of your pockets for a little extra balance.

- **Start slow.** Your body and muscles will take a bit more time to warm up in the cold weather so start out more slowly than you might in warmer weather.

- **Drink up.** You might not feel it, but walking in the dry winter air can be dehydrating, so drink up, before, during, and after your walk.

- **The eyes have it.** The winter sun can be sneaky and snow or ice can magnify what sun there is. Don't head out for a winter walk without a good pair of sunglasses.

- **Everything's better with a friend.** It's always a good idea to walk with a buddy, but even more so in the winter when there may be fewer people around and the risk of falling can be slightly higher.

- **Do less.** If your perfect weather walking typically involves a three-mile loop around the bay, perhaps your cold-weather loop is a mile or two. That's okay: remember, all walking is good walking.

- **Dress for Success.** Layers are your friend, as are wicking fabrics designed to pull moisture away from your skin. Cotton is your enemy, as it tends to hold water and stay damp against your skin. Great accessories are a must, including gloves (or better yet, mittens), a quality hat that covers your ears, warm wool socks, and shoes or boots with sufficient warmth and traction for snow or ice.

If you are prepared for it and acclimated to it, winter walking is awesome. Not acclimated? Not comfortable? Too much snow, wind, and ice? Find yourself a treadmill and keep moving, 'cause all walking is good walking and every mile matters.

Summer Walking: Dog Days of Summer

The first time I visited Arizona was July 1994 during a six-hour layover on the return from a Mexican vacation. I love checking out new places and was excited to spend that six hours exploring Phoenix. I walked out of the airport to find a cab and was struck by the Arizona summer sun. And I mean struck. It was like I stepped into a wall of heat. I stood for a moment thinking my skin was going to melt. Gratefully, I sunk into the first cab that pulled up. "Oh my gosh," I said to the driver, "It is so hot! How do you guys manage?"

He chuckled and said, "Well, you get used to it. We don't spend a lot of time out of doors this time of year and we drink a lot of water. A lot," he motioned to the gigantic bottle of water on the seat beside him.

If cold weather walking provides challenges at one end of the spectrum, hot weather walking provides its own challenges on the other. Once again, our biology is going to work to keep us on the couch because we are wired to avoid taxing our body in the extreme heat. However, we should consider overriding that instruction, but doing so in a careful, thoughtful, and cautious way because, though you can dress and prepare for the cold, there is less to do to make walking in extreme heat safe and comfortable.

So when is it just too hot? That depends on the temperature *and* on the humidity – they combine to impact how our body responds to heat. When it is hot and dry, your body's perspiration works as a natural cooling system – your body cools down as the sweat evaporates from your skin. High humidity means less evaporation and less efficient cooling. As a result, the outdoor temperature doesn't tell the entire story and the "heat index" – which is a measure of temperature and humidity – is a better indicator of when it is safe and comfortable for you to maintain your walking practice. The breeze – or lack of a breeze – plays a part too, as a nice breeze can speed the evaporation of perspiration and help that all-important cooling system.

Other factors come into play, including your overall health, wellness and weight, any underlying health conditions, how well acclimated you are to exercising in the heat, and how strenuous your walk will be.

There are serious risks to pushing yourself too far in too much heat. Heat illness can include everything from dehydration to death. Sometimes, it is just too hot.

But like with cold weather walking, if you take the right precautions, avoid the all-or-nothing mentality, you will still be able to maintain your walking practice most – if not all – days. Here are six things to consider.

1. Shorten it Up. As with cold weather walking, it might be that you need to shorten the duration of your hot summer walks and once again, this is okay. Remember, one mile is infinitely better than zero miles.

2. Dusk and Dawn are your friends. Getting out before the heat of the day takes hold or ending your day with an evening walk is definitely the way to go.

3. Dress for it. While you want clothing that is light and breathable, you also want coverage, especially if you are walking when the sun is up. A hat with a generous brim will help keep the sun from beating down on your head and will help to protect your face and your eyes.

4. Speaking of Your Eyes. Eye protection is essential year round, and especially in the summer when the sun is at its strongest. This protects not just your eyes, but your eyelids, the location for between 5% and 10% of all skin cancers. Since we don't typically put sunblock on our eyes and eyelids, good-quality sunglasses are a must.

5. Water, Water Everywhere. Remember my cab driver. Hydrate before, during, and after.

6. Don't Forget the Sunblock. I know, I know, you know. But we can't be reminded enough. Be sure to get your ears!

When all else fails, when walking outdoors is just not safe or possible, consider mall walking, basement walking, treadmill walking, walking in place because ... and say it with me ... all walking is good walking and every mile matters.

So Many Walks Ways To Walk

Most of us lace up our sneakers (or, depending on where you live, your "tennis shoes", "tennies", or "trainers") and head out for a walk. Same path, same cadence, same intention. And that's great, becoming a creature of habit with your walking goes a long way to helping you maintain that practice. But there's more. More ways to maximize your walking practice. More ways to enjoy your walking practice.

More ways to walk.

I typically walk one of the same three trails day-after-day. Despite the fact that I'm walking in the same places, I take four different kinds of walks, each of which feeds and fuels me in a different way. Often, I'm able to recognize which kind of walk I need and set my intention accordingly.

A Walk in Silence to Find Peace.

Sometimes, I head out for a walk with no distractions, no agenda, and no specific intention. No music. No podcast. No company. It is time to let my mind wander, daydream, and just be. Nothing particular on my mind, no problem I'm seeking to solve. These are the walks that rejuvenate me when I've been working – and thinking – hard and are perfect when I am feeling stressed or overwhelmed. They help me recharge my batteries, repair decision fatigue, fuel up my creativity, and tamp down cortisol – the stress hormone that makes me feel anxious.

They are also the perfect style of walk when there is something lurking at the edge of my mind that needs attention, anxiety I need to understand, feelings, emotions, or grief that I need to process. These are the walks that give my mind, heart, and soul the space they need to do their most important work.

A Walk to Solve Problem

Sometimes, I set out on a walk with the hope of solving a particular problem, processing a particular challenge, or sorting through a particular emotion. Before I leave, I identify exactly what it is that I want to focus on throughout my walk.

As I walk, I think about the issue at hand, and gently bring my mind back when it wanders, which it often does. In this way, these walks become an exercise in mindfulness and attention. Like many people, my brain works best while I'm walking and this tactic has enabled me to find breakthroughs when I've been stuck and generate fresh ideas when I've needed to solve a particularly thorny challenge.

The key is to capture any ideas that arise quickly, before they get lost in the whirlwind of my return to home or office. So, while I walk, I will sometimes record my thoughts and ideas as audio notes in my phone or write them down immediately upon returning home.

A Walk to Lose Myself

Sometimes, I simply want to move my body and lose myself in music or a podcast or a story. These walks are best when I have nothing much on my mind and are especially good if I want to try to rack up the miles and fire up my endorphins. I choose a favorite playlist or podcast and GO. These are the walks that, by the end, have me dancing down the trail singing aloud, or doing an entire second lap because I'm dying to hear how the story ends.

A Walk with Others

Often, I walk with others. As we will explore shortly, it is the best way I know to connect with those I love and those I'm just getting to know.

Free of distractions, out in nature, conversations flow easily from one subject to the next. We connect in a deep way and reap the benefits of sharing the experience of time spent in nature. And wow, the time goes fast when we are walking and talking.

Walker? Hiker? Tomato, Tomato?

Yesterday, instead of walking my typical two-mile dirt road that starts behind the golf course, I decided to try a different trail through the woods. Marked by blue trail markers nailed above eye level on the trees, this three-mile loop starts at a small parking area off of a busy road. It winds through the woods with a few moderate ups and downs, but is never more than a mile from the road and only at the farthest point was I beyond the sound of the occasional truck.

Was I walking or hiking yesterday? For that matter, is my usual walk down the dirt road a walk or a hike?

Walk? Hike? Is there a real distinction or is this merely a *"you say tomato, I say tomato"* situation? Does it matter?

The Difference Between a Walk and a Hike ... at Least in the US

While there is no official distinction, the two words are generally used to describe two different activities, though there is a whole lotta' gray in between.

Generally, at least in the United States, *"hiking"* refers to a relatively long walk on a trail in the countryside taken for pleasure. *"Walking"* refers to a relatively shorter walk in places other than the "countryside" – think walking through your neighborhood or down a city street – for the purpose of getting from one place to the other. So there are two elements to the distinction between walking and hiking: first, the location and second, the intention.

Walking off-road in the countryside for pleasure = hiking.

Walking on-road for the purpose of getting from one place to another = walking.

What constitutes "long" and "the countryside" are obviously open to interpretation, hence oodles of gray area. But it is the "for pleasure" part which I believe is key and goes to the intention of your walk. Is your goal to get from here to there? Are you walking to the neighborhood coffee shop for a morning latte? If *intention* is the key, then what about walking for fitness and wellness? Where does that fit in?

Is my typical walk down a rarely traveled dirt road a "walk" or a "hike"? How 'bout yesterday's 3-mile loop in the woods?

Trying to fit your walking practice into a box of "walk" or "hike" is often impossible and since all walking is good walking, whether you are walking around your suburban neighborhood, hoofing it through the mall to beat the midday heat, or spending the day scaling Mt. Washington, does it *really* matter?

Maybe. The two words do provide a helpful framework to consider how you define yourself and that definition can open your mind to exploring new places.

Let's call yesterday's three-mile trek through the woods a hike. That makes me someone who hikes. Yup, I'm a hiker. Someone who walks in nature for the experience of it.

Once you define yourself as a walker *and* a hiker, new opportunities open. Hikers explore new places. Hikers hike for challenge and pleasure. Hikers are willing to invest in gear to enhance their sport – trekking poles, hiking shoes, clothing designed for varying weather, awesome hiking socks.

Take your walking practice off road, consider yourself a hiker, and oh the places you will go.

A final note. These distinctions don't necessarily apply in other countries. For instance, in much of Europe, a walk could easily refer to a 10-kilometer trek through the Alps, so if someone in Switzerland invites you for a Sunday afternoon "walk," you'd be advised to ask a few questions before you commit.

The Joy of Flânerie

Americans tend to be hard-charging. Data tells us that we work a lot. According to the Organisation for Economic Cooperation and Development, Americans work substantially more hours each year than Germans, Danes, Austrians, and most other Europeans. In fact, in 2020, Americans worked an average of 1,767 while our French counterparts clocked an average of merely 1,402 hours. That gives our French friends 365 hours each year – a full hour each day – to do other things.

It's no wonder that France is the home of the flâneur.

A flâneur is a person who embraces the joy of the wander, the pleasure of a leisurely afternoon stroll or a long walk through the city streets. Without destination, without apparent goal, she wanders.

A flâneur is one who engages in flânerie, which Merriam Webster defines as "aimless or idle quality or state." Aimless. Idle.

I think they got it wrong. A bit more digging reveals that flânerie is far more nuanced. It is not simply the act of aimless wandering, which makes it sound like a waste of time. There's another, more subtle element: flânerie provides the opportunity for exploration and observation that can only be fully experienced when you set out with eyes wide open and the freedom to go where your feet lead. The essence of flânerie is the art of observation and the chance to take in the sounds, the sights, the smells, and the people.

There is huge value in wandering. Heading out without a goal or purpose, allowing ourselves the time and the space to be fully present for whatever moments and experiences present themselves. The richness of the world comes clear when we wander and observe and, consciously or not, we gain a deeper understanding of the world around us.

Though I didn't have the word for it, I was something of a flâneur for the dozen years I lived in New York City. Many Sunday afternoons I would head out onto the city streets without purpose or destination. I would choose a direction and go, often for hours. I explored nooks and crannies of the city, neighborhoods I hadn't known existed. I remember how the smells were different in different neighborhoods, Little Italy versus Chinatown, the Korean dumpling houses on 32nd street, and the Indian spice shops in Murray Hill. Those walks gave me a unique, intimate understanding of my city, and the people who inhabited it. Even now, 25 years later, I can call to memory the exact feel of the pavement beneath my feet.

Coddiwomple

I recently discovered a word: coddiwomple. It is British slang that means "to travel in a purposeful manner towards a vague destination." It is used as both a fact – as applied to a walk – and as a metaphor – as applied to a life. As someone who loves a goal and a plan, who *believes* in the power of goals and plans, I love the concept of coddiwomple and I love how much fun it is to say. Yet I had trouble wrapping my head around it. Can you walk in a purposeful way without a clear destination? Can you work your way through a life of purpose without clear goals?

I've come to decide that you can. Actually, I've come to realize that you probably are.

For the past several years, I have led a weekly walking class that is heard by thousands. During the 30-minute class, I lead my students through a warm-up, various pace changes, and a variety of walking-related exercises. Sometimes the classes have themes – "strut like a model day" is always a favorite – and like most instructors, I've adopted certain phrases that I tend to use over and over again. One of those phrases goes something like this:

> I invite you to walk with purpose. This is not your stroll-ing down the street, letting your dog stop to sniff every bush, pace. This is not your window shopping pace. This is your walking-as-if-you-have-someplace-important-to-go pace. Because you do.

The intention of this instruction is not to help my students define a goal, but rather a style of walking. I'm not telling them where to go, I'm telling them how to move during our time together. In a sense, in virtually every class, I am encouraging my students to coddiwomple.

Be present. Move with purpose. Hold the destination loosely.

Because here's the truth: despite all of our planning, all of our lists, all of the dreams we dream for ourselves, our lives are littered with uncertainty, with both unforeseen challenges and unanticipated opportunities present-ing themselves along the way. Confronted with that reality, we have two choices. We can choose to meander through life, as if we are wandering down the street window shopping. Or we can walk with purpose as if we have someplace important to go – because we do – despite the knowledge that the ultimate destination remains unknown.

I vote we choose to coddiwomple.

Walking with a Beginner's Mind

Remember Claudia Beeney, the highly creative founder of the House of Shine we met earlier? Claudia walks the same path each day, noticing the seasons, the weather, and other subtle changes.

I do much the same thing. I have three trails I typically walk, two in the winter and one in the summer – my "winter trails" get super buggy in the summer, while my "summer trail" tends to be too windy in the winter. Sometimes I change it up and I love to explore new places by foot, but on the day-to-day, I tend to hit the same paths over and over. I've come to appreciate how this enables me to do two things. First, because my feet know the way, my mind is free to wander: I do my most creative thinking while walking these well-worn paths.

There is another, more subtle opportunity that presents itself when you regularly walk in the same place: the chance to practice what Zen Buddhism refers to as Shoshin, or the beginner's mind.

The beginner's mind is the power of coming to each experience with openness and leaving your preconceived notions at the door. This is much harder than it sounds. We have a tendency to not only continue doing things the way we've done them in the past, but to assume, without even thinking about it, that the way we've done them is the "right way" or the "best way" and not worth reconsidering. The more expert or proficient we become, the more our minds tend to close to new ideas or new ways.

Consider how you tie your shoes. Have you ever stopped to contemplate whether or not there is a better way? Probably not. You've probably been tying your shoes the exact same way for decades. And yet over the past few years, new shoe tying methods have begun to spring up, with popular athletic shoes offering a variety of new methods. Are they better? Maybe, maybe not. Or should I say maybe knot ...

Anyway, the point is this ... when we approach problems and situations with a beginner's mind, we have the chance to see opportunities and solutions that we would otherwise miss.

What does this have to do with walking the same trails over and over? Everything. Nurturing and developing your own beginner's mind takes practice and your favorite walk on your favorite trail is a fantastic way to do that.

How?

Take a moment on every walk to see with a fresh eye, as if you'd never walked that path before. Notice – really notice – how every day, that well-loved trail looks and feels different. What color is the sky? Are there buds on the trees in early spring or a hint of red tinging the edges of the leaves in early fall? Can you hear the sound of your feet greeting the ground? Can you feel the air against your skin? And how exactly does your body feel at the start, middle, and end of your walk?

Every walk presents an opportunity to hone the powerful practice of walking through life with a beginner's mind.

Walking as Meditation

I am convinced that meditation is good for you. I've read the articles and listened to the stories from friends and experts who credit their calm and focus to their daily meditation practice.

And I've tried. Four different meditation apps. Three different meditation classes. One long weekend retreat. I've told myself that meditation is a form of mental exercise that I should do even when I don't feel like it. Occasionally, I've even managed to transport myself to a place where I feel like I'm outside of my body, observing my thoughts and letting them float away like clouds.

But mostly, as I sit still, legs crossed on a couch, chair, or cushion, I'm itching to get moving. It's not that I can't sit still and follow my breath, it's that I don't want to.

Instead, walking is my meditation. Walking in silence, in nature, the rhythm of putting one foot in front of the other is what enables me to release control of my thoughts and be fully present.

Turns out, I didn't invent this idea. Yael Shy, a meditation teacher and founder of Mindfulness Consulting, exudes the kind of calm that feels perfect for someone sharing the wisdom of meditation. Over the course of several conversations, she explained that walking meditation finds its roots in Buddhism. "While many of us are familiar with seated meditation, there are actually five postures for meditation in the Buddhist tradition," she explains. "Seated, standing, lying down, kneeling, and walking: Walking meditation is right there at the core of the tradition." Called kinhin, walking meditation offers the chance to become aware and present in movement. "Some people are kinesthetic learners who benefit from feeling things in their bodies," Yael explains.

She is not alone in embracing the benefits of walking meditation. Thich Nhat Hanh, the Vietnamese monk who many credit with helping to popularize meditation and mindfulness, taught about the power of walking to provide a powerful forum for meditation and about the unique way walking meditation can connect us with the earth. In a beautiful poem on walking, he writes:

> *Take my hand.*
> *We will walk.*
> *We will only walk.*
> *We will enjoy our walk*
> *without thinking of arriving anywhere.*

As you head out to explore walking meditation, Yael has some advice. "Begin by placing your attention on one thing, perhaps the bottom of your foot. Once you are in a concentrated place, slowly open up that concentration to your whole body. Remember, you are striving to be not just in your thoughts, but in your experience."

Not just in your thoughts, but in your experience.

Crap. Now that I think about it, I realize that I spent most of my walking time lost in my thoughts. Looks like I still have some work to do on this walking meditation thing. But I suppose they don't call it a practice for nothing.

Play a Walking Game

My parents used to live in a neighborhood that abutted a golf course. Many afternoons, my dad would pedal his bike out of the garage and head down the street to the edge of the development and hunt for wayward golf balls which he would drop into a little bag affixed to the handlebars. Some days, he'd end his hunt empty handed, but other days he would scoop up two, three, and sometimes four golf balls and he would return home, triumphant and sweaty, from what came to be known in the family as "golf-ball hunting." Over time, he acquired a huge box of abandoned golf balls which he donated to a charitable organization that is meaningful to him.

Years went by and my parents moved to a home in a community with no neighboring golf course. Dad needed a new game, so he created one based on the animals he spotted while out walking. Squirrels were worth two points, little lizards were worth three points, and catching a glimpse of a big lizard up on his hindquarters? Five points! While he walked, he kept his attention focused and the tally running in his head. When he returned home, he'd make a note of the date and score in a little notebook.

Sounds silly? Nope, like so much of what my dad does instinctively, it was brilliant. Here's why.

First, dad's games kept his attention focused. His mind wasn't wandering off to his to-do list or things that were stressing him. His focus was right there and he was fully present. In this way, without taking a course or reading a book about it, he was regularly and naturally practicing a powerful form of mindfulness. In essence, my dad gamified mindfulness.

Second, by keeping track of his animal-spotting score, or watching his collection of golf balls grow, he was giving himself tangible motivation to keep going. With every golf ball, dad gave himself a tiny dose of dopamine – which you'll remember can serve as our body's natural motivator, the tiny drip of feel good hormone that encourages us to take that action again and again.

Turning your walk into a mindfulness practice while simultaneously creating a mechanism that encourages you to do it again tomorrow?

Brilliant.

The possible games you can play while you walk are limited only by your imagination, where you live, and what you love. But here are a few ideas to spark your walking game creativity.

- **Color of the Day.** Each day, hunt for something of a specific color. Grab a picture of it. You'll be amazed at the things you'll notice.

- **Letter of the Day.** Same idea ... work your way through the alphabet and each day, strive to spot something that starts with that letter. Snap a photo ... or not.

- **The Weirdest Thing I Saw Today on My Walk Was.** Each day, look for the most unusual thing you can find. Maybe it is a wayward flip flop, or a leaf shaped like a perfect heart.

- **Make Up A Story.** Choose a person, a home, a tree – anything really – and tell yourself a story about it. Make it as rich in detail as possible. Bonus points for writing the story down in a journal when you get home (perhaps one day it could become a book).

- **Look for Awe.** Earlier, we talked about awe walks and the research that teaches that we can often discover awe on our walks simply by looking for it. As you head out on your walk, challenge yourself to find one moment of awe along the way.

- **Count the Animals.** Take a page from my dad's playbook: assign number points for each animal you spot and keep track of your daily animal score.

Get Started. Keep Going.

We know we should. We want to. We long to realize the benefits of an intentional walking practice. But we are busy. So, so busy. We work. We raise families. We say yes, even when we probably should say no. We put too much on our plates and anything remotely resembling self-care gets pushed, over and over again, to the bottom of the list. And when we have time, or have the opportunity to make time, we are tired. We don't feel like it. Sometimes it is too cold, sometimes it is too hot. Sometimes it rains. But mostly, we just don't feel like it.

Getting started and keeping going should be easy. But it's not.

Why is it so hard to do something that we know will make us feel better physically and mentally? Why don't we crave movement, exercise, and *walking* with as much zeal as we crave coffee, ice cream, or a foot massage?

Our bodies are biologically and evolutionarily wired to conserve energy, encouraging us to move as little as possible in case we need that energy to outrun a sabertooth tiger or outlast a famine.

Apparently, our minds aren't much help either.

Dr. Laurie Santos is a Professor of Psychology at Yale University and host of the popular podcast *The Happiness Lab*. She has made a deep study of human happiness and has concluded that our minds are not very good at telling us what will make us happy.

"There's lots of evidence that we don't always do the things that we know are good for our well being," she told me when I posed the question to her. "Often there's a disconnect between what we know we need to do and what we do." Like walking, which Dr. Santos agrees, is one such practice. "There's lots of evidence that exercise can really improve symptoms of depression and even anxiety and improve our happiness, that walking with other people gives us the chance to be social and that social connection is the kind of thing that can improve our well-being over time. Finally, when people walk, they pay attention and are mindful about their environment and there's lots of evidence that being present can really improve your well-being over time."

Against the backdrop of lives that have become perhaps too busy, and complicated by the fact that we might not "feel" like going for a walk, even when it is precisely what our minds, our moods, or our bodies need, how do we build and maintain an intentional walking practice?

Start Where You Are. Not Where They Are, Where You Are.

First things first: you need to let go of expectations and start where you are. This requires you to be honest with yourself. Sounds obvious, right? But in our compare and despair culture, where social media coaxes us to compare ourselves to others, many have a tendency to look at what someone else is doing and think that is what we are supposed to be doing. We are not.

Do you have any injuries or illnesses that would make it wise to consult a doctor before starting any new exercise program? Are you someone who hits the gym four days a week and wants to add a walking practice to your life for the added movement, mobility, and mental benefits? Have the last dozen years seen you commuting an hour to work, sitting behind your computer all day before commuting another hour home? Are you in the throes of a depression that makes the mere act of leaving your house feel daunting and overwhelming? Were you a college athlete who hasn't moved since she last hung up her field hockey stick so, while you still have the heart of an athlete, your body has not kept up? Are you carrying more weight than is optimal, dealing with injuries or illness? Right this moment, are you home in Alaska in January or Arizona in August? Are you the caregiver for an infant, aging parent, or sick spouse?

Being honest with ourselves can be hard. Starting where we are can feel discouraging. But it is the only way.

Then, Set Your Own Goal

Once you've gotten honest, it is time to set a goal, 'cause we humans love goals. Working towards a specific goal in small, tangible steps that you can accomplish (as opposed to setting goals you can't) puts your dopamine encouragement system to work for you. So if you are trying to create a regular walking practice, start with a goal. A reasonable "Goldilocks Goal," one that is achievable yet ambitious. Challenging, but possible.

If 10,000 steps a day isn't the gold standard for everyone, and we've already talked about all of the reasons why it isn't, what *is* the right goal? Should we count steps, miles, or minutes? Do hills matter? If I can't go as fast or as far as my sister Susie or neighbor Dora, should I even bother? What about the days when I'm tired, or injured or just too friggin' busy to do what I typically do?

How do I set a walking goal and, for that matter, should I even bother?

Let's consider the last question first: should I even bother setting a goal when I know weather, circumstances, *life*, is likely to disrupt my plans and alter my course? Yes. Absolutely. Setting goals, knowing that they may change, can make your life richer, fuller, and help insure that you are putting your time and energy towards the things that matter most. And yes, sure, this is about setting your walking goal, but it is about so much more.

Let's say you are setting sail on a big and epic journey, perhaps crossing the Atlantic from England to New York. In a sailboat. Before you set sail, you precisely target your destination and carefully plot your course. Yet you know that storms will pull you off course along the way, forcing you to readjust your sails and reset your headings. Knowing those storms are likely to come, do you set out without bothering to identify your destination or set your course? Of course not. That would be insane.

That's the power of setting a goal. We need to choose our destination and chart our course. And when the storms come, and they will, we need to be ready to batten down the hatches and adjust the sails as needed. Because, as Yogi Berra put it, *"if you don't know where you are going, you might wind up someplace else."*

How do you set that goal? It is so, so easy to just take the 10,000-step goal that the industrial fitness complex, media, and connected devices have been shoving down our throats for decades. Who has time to be introspective or to figure out the goal that works best for them?

You do. And here's the secret: if you set your own goal, research has shown that you are more likely to achieve it.

Researchers from the University of Pennsylvania sought to determine the most effective goal-setting strategy to encourage physical activity among 500 individuals at risk for heart attack. Some of the study's participants were assigned a specific number for the number of daily steps they should accomplish, while others were allowed to set their own daily step goals. Sure enough, those who were permitted to set their own goals and immediately got to walking were the only group to show significant improvements in daily physical activity levels.

If setting your own goal is key to your success, how do you find a goal that works?

First, you need to be objective and clear about where you are starting and the challenges you will confront as you build your walking practice. Have you been sedentary for the past many years? Are you managing an illness or injury? If so, the best place to start is with the advice of a doctor. While walking is generally safe for most, and often the first step (pun intended) toward recovery, a doctor's advice is important.

If you're in generally good health and tend to move throughout your day comfortably, start with an honest assessment of your abilities and time. Can you manage a 10-minute walk after dinner three days each week? Awesome. A 2-mile walk through the woods twice each week? Great. Both? You go! Here are a few goals set by members of our walking community over the years:

- I will walk the ½ mile down the driveway to get my mail rather than drive unless it is snowing or raining too hard;
- I will walk while my daughter is in gymnastics class;
- I will walk 50 intentional miles each month;
- I will set up a weekly "walk and talk" with my friend Stacy every Tuesday morning at 8:00.

Setting a goal that is reasonable, achievable but still ambitious is the key to your success.

Two Ways to Keep Going: Build a Walking Habit. Or Don't.

Once you've taken that first step and set that goal, the question becomes: what can you put in place to help you achieve it? Below, I will explore two approaches. The first is to build a walking *habit*. The second is to become what I call an "opportunistic walker."

Importantly, these two options are not mutually exclusive. You can both build a walking habit and be an opportunistic walker and, if at all possible, you should.

Let's explore.

Put Habits to Work For You

For years while my daughter was in high school, I had a very set routine. Before I went to bed at night, I'd place the next day's exercise clothes in a basket in the bathroom. In the morning, I'd stumble into the bathroom at about 5:20 and reach for them. By 5:30, my teeth were brushed and I was dressed for my walk. There was no thinking, planning, or debating. I'd spend the next 90 minutes sipping coffee, doing my morning routine, making lunches, and working.

At 7:00, I'd step out onto the front porch with my daughter to wait for the school bus, which she'd board right around 7:05. I'd wave as the bus pulled away and immediately start walking. If I walked back into the house, if I sat down to answer a single email, I'd be sunk. But if I kept going with that routine, that habit, my walk would be done by 8:00 am. A happy habit.

Habits can work both ways. We can create habits that serve us and those that don't. Here was one of my other habits.

At 3:00, I'd get home from the office and walk in the front door to wait for my daughter to get off the bus. That was my cue.

I'd go directly to the kitchen and open the pantry to pull out nuts or chips or cookies, then I'd sit back down at my computer for one last check of my email while I snacked mindlessly waiting for her to come crashing through the door. That was my routine.

I got to crunch on something salty or sweet. That was my reward.

Mindlessly snacking while I waited for my daughter to get off the bus was a habit that didn't serve my goals and one which, unfortunately, I executed on most days with very little thought.

Entire books have been written about habits. Developing new positive habits and changing old negative habits is not easy, even if you understand the formula. But understanding the basic mechanics of habits is a good place to start.

Boatloads of research, including an extensive study from MIT which is described in *The Power of Habit*, have revealed two important things about habits.

First, habits have three distinct components: (1) the trigger or cue; (2) the routine; and (3) the reward. Understanding this is helpful because it provides a framework by which we can alter our habits – either encourage good ones or discourage bad ones – by changing these clearly defined elements.

Second, habits light up a different part of our brain than our more thoughtful actions and we execute them largely on auto-pilot.

This helps because it means that once we ingrain a positive habit, we are far more likely to replicate it without having to talk ourselves into it each and every time.

The bad news is that habits are tricky, tricky things. New positive cues take time to cultivate while cues that trigger negative routines can't always be avoided: while my daughter was in school, I always walked into my house at about 3:00. Since so many of our habits happen on auto-pilot, it takes a lot of mindfulness to change them.

Creating a new habit is easier than obliterating an old. One effective tactic is to replace a "bad" habit with a "good" habit you'd like to foster. For instance, it proved to be easier to replace my afternoon snack with a new habit than to simply keep doing everything the same way – walk in the door, sit down at the computer, but will myself not to get the snack.

I decided to try to replace my snacking habit with a ten-minute dog walk.

I began by hanging Moose's leash on the door before I left for work: the new cue.

I decided a ten-minute walk around the block was the habit I'd strive to cultivate: the new routine.

I observed that after the walk, I felt refreshed, energized, and had forgotten about the snack: the new reward.

After about a week, I discovered that not only had I begun to create a new habit for myself, I had created a habit for my dog: when I walk in the door after work (the cue) he expects a walk (the routine) and when we get home, he is happy (the reward).

Apparently, dogs are creatures of habit as well.

Habits often evolve through the things that we do on repeat. But they can be created intentionally. Where in your life can you add a walking habit? A ten-minute walk after the dinner dishes are done? A morning walk before work? A lunchtime walk with a friend? An evening walk before bed? A Sunday morning walk with your partner? A walking group that meets Tuesdays and Thursdays?

Be Opportunistic

Creating a walking habit is great. But so is being an opportunistic walker, one who looks for – and takes advantage of – slices of time that present opportunities to move.

It was 3:30 and I realized I had been sitting in front of my computer since just before 8:00 that morning. My eyes were glazing over, but I still had six tasks left on my to-do list for the day. However, none of them were time-sensitive and no deadlines lurked. The sun was shining. I had to pick my daughter up from field hockey practice at 4:30. I had an hour. 60 minutes. I got up, changed into my favorite sneakers, and walked out the door.

I am an opportunistic walker. I look for windows of opportunity in my day and when one opens and the thought *"I could take a walk"* crosses my mind, I act on it. I try not to overthink it and I don't talk myself out of it. If my mind goes to *"well, I should ...."* clean the kitchen, start dinner, answer one more email, weed the garden ... I shut those thoughts down and walk out the door.

Chances are, there are windows that will open in your life. Moments when you feel anxiety that could be ameliorated by a walk, when the crisp fall air beckons, when a meeting gets canceled, or when you complete a project earlier than expected. You can fill that time with a thousand tasks because there will always be one more email to answer, a bathroom to clean, another bill to pay, or a window that could stand to be washed. Or, you can take that opportunity to do the thing that can transform your mind, mood, and body: take a walk.

Find a Friend, or Five

This is one of my favorite texts to receive: "Wanna walk at 4:30?" I have four different friends who send that, or similar texts, to me on a regular basis. My personal policy is simply this: if I don't have anything on my calendar that absolutely, positively prevents me from saying yes, then I say yes. Because I know that walking with friends checks four boxes at one time: I get to be in nature. I get exercise. I get the physical, mental, and emotional benefits of a walk. And I get to spend quality, undistracted time with a friend.

Often, I'm the one who sends the text. If you haven't created a small group of friends who motivate you off the couch by texting you to join them for a walk – what do you do? Where do you start?

It's simple. Just start. Today. Text a friend and invite them to take a walk with you. Some will say yes, others will say no. You will probably need to keep asking and inviting at least for a while. But then – and here is the key – they will begin to ask you. And when they do, say yes.

Dogs Help, Too

His name was Kibo. I remember the day we chose his name. Eric and I were laying on the bed in his apartment with a huge atlas spread out in front of us. "Denali?" He offered. "Bryce?" I countered. We went back and forth like that for a while. "Kibo, the highest point on Mt. Kilimanjaro," one of us – I don't remember which – suggested. And that was it. Days later we picked up the six-pound Portuguese Water Dog puppy who would grow up to be a therapy dog who worked weekly with disabled adults, a water rescue dog who life-guarded our children without ever being taught to do so, and the best friend to every member of our family. He was the dog of dogs. When he was nearing the end of his life, cancer taking him from us way too soon, my parents flew up from Florida to say goodbye. His picture still sits in my office, and talking about him invariably brings both a smile to my face and a tear to my eye.

During our decade or so together, we walked. Every day at about 11:00, he came into the office and asked to walk to the coffee shop where there was always a biscuit waiting for him. We walked through the neighborhood and down to the beach. We drove to the mountains and hiked together. We walked in the woods so many times I can't begin to count them.

Dogs help. Having a dog has been associated with a greater likelihood of heart attack survival, lower blood pressure, triglyceride, and cholesterol levels and better emotional, psychological, and cardiovascular health.

According to a 2019 study by researchers at the University of Liverpool, dog owners walked almost 200 minutes more each week than their non-canine owning neighbors and were four times as likely to meet or exceed the recommended physical activity guidelines. Not only that, but children living with dogs showed "greater participation in recreational walking and free time physical activity."

Perhaps even more interesting – and somewhat unexpected – dog owners spent more time than the non-dog owners engaging in other forms of physical activity without their dogs. The researchers concluded that, "dog owners are considerably more active than people without a dog, and that dog walking is undertaken in addition to, and not instead of, other physical activities."

That said, the study didn't show cause and effect, but rather correlation. Perhaps more active people simply choose to get a dog. But I don't believe it, and neither does Kate.

Last week, walking one of my favorite dirt road trails, I ran into Kate and her husband. Having not seen each other for quite a while, we stopped to chat and, as conversations with me often do, the conversation turned to walking. "We're without a dog for the first time in decades and I just haven't been walking as much," Kate bemoaned. "I'm finding it so much harder to push myself to get out the door."

I hear that. When I walk in the door at about 3:00, Moose goes crazy. He spins in circles by the front door, barking, unable to contain his excitement. Trying to explain to him all of the reasons why we can't walk today, or why I don't want to walk today (it's raining, it's cold, I still have work to do, I have to start dinner) does nothing to dissuade him. It is like having a combination of an insistent toddler and accountability coach wrapped up in one happy, bouncy, barky little package.

Yes, Moose, I'm coming.

How to Keep Going

For some people, starting a new practice is hard. Perhaps a voice in their head says, *"You've tried before and failed, so why bother?"* Maybe they are so deep in the routines of their lives that there doesn't feel like there is room to add anything else. Maybe they don't know where to start, are afraid of change, or don't really want to do the thing, but they feel like they "should." Or maybe any one of a dozen other things stop them from getting started.

For others, getting started is the easy part. A new challenge or the promise of transformation is enough to send them shopping for the right gear, setting their alarm, and heading out the door at dawn. For them, the challenge is to keep going.

"I've started so, so many times," sighs my friend, Kindra. "I've tried indoor cycling and yoga and I've joined three different gyms. After a few weeks, I give up."

She's not alone: study after study shows that the vast majority of people who start a new exercise program quit within just a few months. Quitting even happens when things seem to be going well, when we are walking several times a week and experiencing all of the benefits. We feel better. We have more energy. We are happier. Our doctor exclaims how much our "numbers" improved and when she asks us what we are doing, we proudly say, "Walking," and she says, "Well, keep it up, it's working."

And then. Then something happens and we lose our way. We get the flu, sprain an ankle, or the dreaded plantar fasciitis settles in. Maybe we add an extra shift at work to help make a car payment, or one of our kids gets sick, or ... maybe we just get bored.

And don't even get me started talking about winter in Minnesota.

Despite your best intentions, things will conspire to get in the way of your walking practice.

It may be that something deeper is holding you back from accomplishing the things you set out to accomplish, making the changes you need to make, or grabbing hold of the life you want. Once again, therapy might help. But so might simple tactics that you can employ to keep yourself on track or trail.

The Only-When-You-Walk-Book, Playlist, or Podcast

Here's something most people don't know about me: I love crappy, sappy television, page-turning mysteries and serial podcasts, where the story unfolds episode by episode.

If this is you, there is a simple tactic you can leverage to help you stick to your walking practice. Designate an audio book, a podcast, or a special playlist your "walk only" entertainment.

The rule is very simple: you listen to it only when you are walking.

Ask Yourself: What Can I Do?

For three long years, I wrestled with a lower-back injury. There were days when every breath sent pain ricocheting down my back, and entire nights when spasms kept me awake. It was awful.

It would come and go and there were stretches of time when things seemed okay. I walked a few miles with my friends on my favorite wooded trails, walked Moose, went into the gym and gingerly lifted weights, far lighter than I had in the past. More than a dozen times, just when I thought I was getting better, I would do something that sent me back to Advil and ice. It was frustrating and, frankly, scary. Would I ever be able to move without pain? Was I always going to feel like I had to hold back and be careful? Would I be afraid to tie my shoes or pick up the laundry basket forever?

There was a day when everything began to change. I had been feeling good and had gone into the gym with a plan. Within minutes, I moved in a way that made my back scream, "Not today!" Nothing I had planned for that little workout was going to be possible. There would be no sit-ups, no rowing, and no squats. I was angry, frustrated, and discouraged. I grabbed my bag and slammed out the door. But then I stopped, literally mid-step, and asked myself, "Okay, what can I do?"

What can I do?

That has become a mantra for me. When the world disrupts my plans, whatever they are, I pause and ask myself *what can I do?*

There's thunder and lightning and it's not safe to walk outside.

What can I do?

My friend Annmarie just canceled our walk because of a work emergency.

What can I do?

Dad is sick and I need to cancel everything and fly to Florida to help.

What can I do?

I'm too tired to do the two-mile walk I had planned, I don't have time to drive to the park where I was planning to walk, my son has a fever …

What can I do?

Because here's the thing: there is usually something you can do, some small step you can take toward whatever goal you are chasing. Maybe you have ten minutes, or five minutes, or maybe you can just walk up and down the stairs in your house a few times.

Ask yourself "what can I do" and then remind yourself that it all counts.

Hack a Human Wiring Flaw and Find an Accountability Partner

I've always believed there is a flaw in the way we humans are wired: we are more likely to show up for others than we are for ourselves. If we commit to meeting a friend for a walk, we are far less likely to skip than if we simply tell ourselves, *"I will walk this afternoon."* Perhaps that's not really a flaw since, as we will explore in the next chapter, we are social creatures and keeping the commitments we make to others helps to strengthen those very important bonds. Nevertheless, it seems to me that we should value the commitments we make to ourselves at least as highly as we value those we make to others. But we don't.

That said, we can hack that tendency to help keep ourselves moving forward. We talked about the effectiveness of planning walking dates with friends and you can take that one step further by finding yourself an accountability partner.

"You're in the midst of writing a book too?" I asked.

"Yes, I'm about halfway through the first draft and this is when it gets hard," Lisa replied. She had invited me to be a guest on her podcast and we were having our pre-podcast, getting-to-know-you call.

"I hear you," I said. At the time, I was midway through the writing of this very book and I was feeling stuck. Other things had taken priority and my writing had stalled. "What's your timeline?" I asked.

"I'm hoping to have a draft done by the end of the year," she said. It was May.

"Me too!" I was excited that there was someone else on my timeline, confronting similar struggles. "We could be accountability partners," I suggested.

"Yes! I would love that," Lisa said.

An accountability partner is someone with whom you have shared your goal and with whom you check in on a regular basis with your progress. It can be reciprocal: you can help them stay on track with their goal in much the same way they help you.

The ideal accountability partner is someone you trust and with whom you can be honest: if you are tempted to exaggerate your progress, the relationship won't work. Your accountability partner is part cheerleader, reminding you that you can keep going when the going gets tough, and delivers just the right amount of tough love, reminding you to keep going when excuses creep in. Whether you touch base with your accountability daily or weekly, a consistent cadence on communication is key. Finally, your accountability partner has to take your goals seriously and, if the relationship is reciprocal, you have to commit to helping them achieve their goals as well.

Embrace the Work and Notice the Incremental Changes

Looking for an instant fix to all that is wrong in your life? Hoping to defeat depression, lose 72 pounds, and beat cancer? Walking can help, sure. But it's not going to help by itself and it's not going to help overnight.

We have been taught to look for instant results. Frankly, I blame the media. So many companies peddle instant transformation if you just buy their potion or sign up for their program. There are few places where this is as blatant as around weight loss, where "before and after" photos are advertising de rigueur.

Pretty much nothing works that way. Pretty much everything of value takes work, time, and consistency. Sometimes for months, often for years.

In order to keep going, you need to embrace the journey, fall in love with the work and celebrate the small, incremental changes. How? That's simultaneously simple and complex.

When you are moving your body, feel your heart pounding just a bit harder in your chest, and notice that trickle of sweat running down the center of your back, embrace the discomfort and remind yourself that you are getting stronger and healthier. Treat the work with love.

When you get back from your walk, pause for a moment to recognize that you feel just a little bit calmer, a little bit happier, a little bit more patient than on the days you don't walk.

Then get up the next day and do it again. And again. Make it a practice, and over time it will become a part of what you do and who you are. It will become your personal practice as it has become mine.

Beat The All or Nothing Mentality

Okay, so at this point, I know you might be thinking "I'm in! I've tried so many programs and made so many commitments before but I get it now – walking is a form of exercise I can do. Starting tomorrow, I'm going to walk every single day, no matter what."

Every single day, no matter what.

And that's the problem. Many of us suffer from an all-or-nothing mentality. We think in absolutes: good or bad. Active or couch potato. Fit or fat. Dieting or binging. I've heard it time and time again, thought it myself, and been told it by my friends: *I missed a day and then it became two, and then five, and I don't know what happened ....*

I know what happened.

First, you broke the habit. Whatever habit or routine you had in place, it broke. Whether by your own doing or something else (weather, injury, illness, travel), your walking routine got off track.

Second, you told yourself, whether consciously or not, that you failed. And, just possibly, your negative voice added the word "again" to that thought, as in *"I thought this time would be different but I failed. Again."*

All or nothing is a story we tell yourselves. But it's not true. Your success or failure, whether with your walking practice or, frankly, anything else in your life, is not going to be the result of one missed day – or even two or even ten. It is going to be the result of your willingness to get up the next day and try again. Fall down seven times and get up eight.

Your walking practice is no different. When the routine is interrupted, there is a simple solution: lace up your sneakers and head out the door. Because as soon as you take one walk, you begin to reinstate that routine and, more importantly, you tell your negative voice that it is wrong. You didn't quit. You didn't give up. This time *is* different. Just one walk changes the story. Just one walk moves you forward.

Chances are, you will have to do this over and over and over because things will happen to pull you off of your walking practice. You will miss days and that is okay. Let me say that again: that is okay. Because we are the kind of people who let the past go. We are the kind of people who move forward, one step at a time.

Part III: The Power of Walking Together

The Power of Walking Together

**"Walking with a friend in the dark is better
than walking alone in the light."**
Helen Keller

"When we walk and talk," says my frequent walking partner Helen, "it's like friendship and bonding and therapy and relationship advice and business development and resource sharing and exercise and fresh air, all rolled into one beautiful walk."

It was the first day of spring, the sun was high in the sky, and we were exploring a new trail in the woods where we often walk together. For years, I've walked with various friends in these woods, talking about every possible topic, from relationships to politics, parenting to menopause, business to religion. We've talked about restaurants we love, trips we've taken, and dreams we've abandoned. We've shared our fears and successes, goals and ideas. You name it, we've talked about it.

In December of 2019, just months before the COVID pandemic shut the world down, I took the stage to deliver a 10-minute talk on the power of walking together to combat loneliness. I began by sharing the surprising results of a survey taken by my company that revealed that more than 72% of the 2,300 women we surveyed regularly experience periods of loneliness. This loneliness is at odds with a deep human drive to connect with others, and study after study has confirmed that meaningful connections are key to both longevity and happiness.

Yet our study revealed another interesting fact: those women who regularly walked with friends were 2.5 times less likely to often experience loneliness.

2.5 times.

That insight piqued my curiosity and launched a journey into the nature of human connection and the physiological, mental, and emotional impact of walking together. Along the way, I met a young Black man who discovered the healing "walk sound" of neighbors walking side-by-side, a mom who created a "walking school bus," a cardiologist who discovered a way to get his patients to finally take the walks he prescribed, a therapist who walked with his young patients, and so, so many others who walk to connect with their loved ones.

I can't wait for you to meet the incredible individuals who have shared their stories of the transformative power of walking together.

Let's go.

Walking as an Antidote to the Loneliness Epidemic

"I feel like I don't have a single close friend in the world." That was the response shared by a woman identified only as Susan P in our survey of 2,300 women. She's not alone.

Much had been written about the loneliness epidemic that was sweeping the country even before the 2020 COVID pandemic drove us deeper into our homes and further away from one another. A report by Harvard University showed that 61% of young adults, 51% of mothers with young children, and 36% of all Americans feel lonely "frequently" or "almost all the time," while a 2020 study by the health insurer Cigna suggests that more than three in five Americans are lonely. Though statistics vary by study, researchers, psychologists, doctors, and social scientists agree: the incidence of loneliness continues to rise.

All of this loneliness comes at a steep cost. Feelings of loneliness have been associated with increases in depression, suicide, dementia, heart disease, anxiety, and premature death. According to Dr. Vivek Murthy, who served as the 19th and 21st Surgeon General of the United States and who is also the author of *Together, The Healing Power of Human Connection in a Sometimes Lonely World*, loneliness is so detrimental to our health and well-being that "loneliness and weak social connections are associated with a reduction in lifespan similar to that caused by smoking 15 cigarettes a day."

15 cigarettes a day.

As human beings, we were not meant to raise our families behind white picket fences at the end of long, isolated driveways. We were meant to live in communities, surrounded by family and friends. This desire for human connection is deeply encoded in our fundamental wiring: our ancestors were a whole lot safer walking through the woods with their tribe than they were wandering alone.

Research, personal experience, and countless anecdotal stories confirm that walking together is a powerful way to build those critical connections and stave off loneliness. Why is that? What is it about walking together that is so good for relationships?

Walking together delivers four things that help form connections and forge relationships. Walking together provides:

- Shared experiences;
- Undistracted time;
- Synchronicity; and
- Better brains and helpful hormones.

Shared Experiences

When my son was 13, we moved from the house in which he had been raised since birth. Though our new home was merely six miles away, it brought us to a new community and, most importantly for him, a new school. While he said the kids were nice, he felt left out. One day, he voiced his feelings about his new classmates. "They have all been together since kindergarten and have all of these shared experiences and memories. I never know what they are talking about."

Fortunately, we had met – and come to like – several of the families and parents of boys in the grade, so I pulled my husband aside and said, "Go make some friggin' memories." And that is how the annual boys rafting trip was born. Every summer from then on, six boys and four dads loaded up their cars and headed off for a weekend of camping and rafting. Experiences were shared, memories were made, and relationships were formed.

Shared experiences are a bedrock of personal connections and research suggests that we enjoy activities more when we share them. A fascinating study from Yale University found that sharing an experience with another person amplifies our perception of that experience. The study was fairly simple and involved chocolate (and any study that involves eating chocolate is, in my mind, a good one).

The researchers separated the subjects into two groups and had them each taste a piece of chocolate with one key difference: in one group, the people were paired up and tasted the chocolate at the same time as their partner, while in the other group each person tasted the chocolate while their partner was looking at a book. The people who tasted the chocolate at the same time as their partners rated the chocolate better tasting. This concept – that sharing an experience with another magnifies how we feel about that experience – means that we are likely to enjoy a walk, and remember it more fondly, when we share it with a friend. That positive association is likely to foster positive feelings towards that friend, deepening our feelings of connection.

Eric and I have been walking together for decades. And that means we have a raft of conversations that begin with "remember" ... *the day we saw the seals frollicking on a walk along the Montauk coast? The walk in Maui when we came up with the idea for our new business? The time we got caught in the rain and the other time we started our walk too late and ended up walking home in the dark? The day we came upon two young children we thought were lost in the woods, but were, instead, the victims of some tough love we didn't fully understand?*

Shared experiences, shared memories, deeper connection.

Check.

Undistracted Time

I remember the night I first answered an email from my bed. I was in a hotel room in New York City following a long day of meetings. Earlier that afternoon, I had bought my first Blackberry, the device that would become ubiquitous among my colleagues until Apple ate the Blackberry.

I pulled the matte black, toast-shaped device out of its box, fired it up, connected my email, and watched in amazement as my inbox filled. I sent my first email to my sister – she had unlocked the magic of the Blackberry just a few weeks before and had inspired me to become an early adopter. "I'm emailing you FROM MY BED," I yelled via email.

And so it began.

It seems almost impossible to believe, but before 2000, less than 28% of Americans had a cell phone and, at that point, cell phones were just phones. Then came email and text messaging and the day I was sitting in my friend Susan's kitchen when she whipped out her phone and shared a photo of her gorgeous guacamole on social media. "You post to Facebook *from your phone*?" I asked, incredulous.

She looked at me funny. "Don't you?"

Fast forward less than two decades and, while these magic little devices have connected us in many ways, research shows they have divided us in many others.

This morning, I went to my local coffee shop to pick up a cup of coffee before heading to the office. In the past, I would have walked in, placed my order, and exchanged pleasantries with the barista while my favorite dark roast brewed. Instead, I placed my order on my phone before getting out of the car, grabbed my coffee from the to-go window and mumbled a vague "thank you" across the shop. No chit chat, no pleasantries, not even a passing comment about the unseasonably cold weather.

Last night, my family sat down to dinner and, though there was no phone in sight, I felt my body tense as I heard text message after text message come in from my husband's gym buddies. Though his phone was tucked in his pocket out-of-sight, I knew that his attention was diverted from my daughter and I, wondering who was texting and what they were saying. And my 20-year-old son? Barely a moment goes by when his attention is fully present and not distracted by the pings and dings of his phone.

All of this digital connectedness is having a significant impact on our relationships.

As early as 2012, researchers discovered that the mere presence of a phone negatively impacted the formation of a relationship. Interested in understanding the consequences of cell phones on things like trust, intimacy, and empathy, the researchers had people sit across from one another and assigned them a topic to discuss. There was one difference: for half of the participants, a phone sat on a nearby table while for the others, a book sat in the same spot. The phone didn't ring, ding, or buzz. Neither participant picked it up. It just sat there. Yet, its mere presence appears to have "inhibited the development of interpersonal closeness and trust, and reduced the extent to which individuals felt empathy and understanding from their partners," and this inhibition appeared to be "most pronounced if individuals were discussing a personally meaningful topic."

And it seems it is just getting worse.

So pervasive is the practice of becoming distracted from the person we are with by our phones that we have created an entirely new word to describe it: phubbing (phone + snubbing). Chances are, you have experienced a time when you were with your partner, friend, colleague or family member when they suddenly appeared to leave the conversation – mentally – and picked up their phone. Yup, you've been phubbed and it doesn't feel good. According to the research, chances are very good that you've done it to others, including to your romantic partner.

Researchers from Baylor University sought to determine just how potentially damaging phubbing – or Partner Phubbing as they called it – can be to our romantic relationships and concluded that our cell phones' frequent interruptions "can undermine our satisfaction with our romantic relationships." No surprise: Partner Phubbing is not conducive to the kind of meaningful conversations and connections that are key to relationship satisfaction.

You know what is? Walking together.

Sure, when you are walking, you can be tracking steps, checking your email, and responding to text messages. But most people don't. I don't know exactly why that is, I just know that it's true. Most people treat a walk, especially an intentional walk in nature, with far more reverence than, say, sitting in a coffee shop together. Thus creating the opportunity for undistracted time walking together.

Synchronicity

It was the early afternoon on the March day the clocks sprang forward. The sun was high in the sky and the thermometer beat 50 for the first time in months. It felt like spring.

I was driving to meet a friend for a walk when I turned the corner and came upon three women walking together in the middle of the road. They were deep in conversation and moving at a good pace. I slowed to a stop to give them the chance to move over to the shoulder and watched the way their feet struck the ground in perfect synchronicity as if they were a marching band that had practiced together for years. Right, left, right, left …

Apparently, this was not a coincidence nor an aberration. When people walk together – despite differences in height, gait or typical walking speed – they have a strong tendency to synchronize their movements and walk at the same pace and in the same rhythm. In what researchers deemed the "first study of synchronized walking," they found that even though the pairs "were never asked to walk synchronously and this was the first time they walked together" they walked as a synchronized unit in almost 50% of all the trials. "This is far above what might be expected by chance – there are an infinite number of combinations of stride lengths and step rates that can produce a given walking speed, and left to chance, two walkers should essentially never synchronize."

And yet we do.

Without speaking, this synchronization provides a sense of connection and unity. Synchronized movement leads to increased cooperative and prosocial behaviors in both adults and children including increased helping, affiliation, bonding, rapport, likeability, and attachment.

And, as we will see in a bit, synchronous movement also helps with conflict resolution.

Right, left, right, left...

Better Brains and Helpful Hormones

As we've discussed, our brains process differently when we are walking. Because part of our brain is occupied putting one foot in front of the other, the rest of our brain is free to roam, to problem solve, think more deeply and creatively – a perfect recipe for meaningful conversation.

In addition, the stress hormone cortisol is reduced, helping us to become more relaxed and focused. And those so-called happy hormones – dopamine, serotonin, and endorphins – fire up. But there's one more hormone that likely becomes relevant when we talk about what happens when we walk together: oxytocin.

Oxytocin heightens our ability to empathize and feel emotions. Research suggests that oxytocin relaxes us, fires up our desire for kinship, makes us care about other people, and encourages us to work together and collaborate. Yes, oxytocin is the same hormone that is triggered during labor and nursing – which makes sense, since it encourages us to bond with our babies.

Walking together is precisely the type of experience that has been shown to increase levels of oxytocin. The combination of a shared experience, physical activity and social interaction can all work together to impact the release of oxytocin, making us feel even more closely connected.

**

Shared experiences. Undistracted time together. Moving in sync and the gift of helpful hormones all working together to make walking together one of the very best ways to create and deepen meaningful relationships.

Walking With Those You Love
Walking with Your Partner: Jennifer's Story

"Our kids are grown, the last one graduated college and moved out last August," Jennifer Farris began when I asked her how her walking practice has impacted her relationship. "Now that they are on to the next phase, there was no excuse and I could fully focus on myself. I went to a doctor and was advised that I needed blood pressure meds and had to lose weight. I realized that I could be in the same place in a year, or I could take charge of my health. That's where my walking journey started.

"My husband and I both have hectic and demanding jobs where we are on the phone and computer all day, frequently on calls, and connected all the time. We do spend a lot of time together, but exercise was something he enjoyed and I didn't. He would go run and I would stay home and read a book. He's always wanted me to go out for walks and runs with him, and I've always said 'I don't have time' or, 'That's not my thing.'

"When I began walking, my husband joined me. It started with one-mile walks and has evolved into weekly Sunday adventures. They are times for us to pause, slow down, put away phones, and spend time together without distractions. We feel closer and, as importantly, I feel healthier, stronger, more energetic, and overall happier. This helps me feel less stressed and more balanced.

"Our weekly Sunday journey is 4.2 miles each way. We walk to our favorite breakfast place, have breakfast, and then walk the 4.2 miles back. Typically on the way there, we have our headphones in and use this time to warm-up, wake-up, and just enjoy being outside. We look for the beauty in nature... the sunrise over the ocean, flowers blooming, birds, and point out whatever we see. It's a leisurely walk often in a comfortable silence.

"On the way home after we've had our coffee and breakfast, we talk about all kinds of things, small things and major life things. We talk about our upcoming week, anything going on with our kids, travel we'd like to do, financial commitments we'd like to make, and future retirement plans. What we don't talk about is work, that is off limits to give ourselves time together without worry or stress of the office. Our Sundays are our special time and we both look forward to. It's an opportunity for us to be active together, be healthier, and relaxed before we start our week. It puts us both in a refreshed state of mind.

"We also take several two or three mile walks during the week. Those are times to release a stressful day, talk about any difficulties we had, clear our heads, and get in a better frame of mind for our evenings together. Scheduling daily time for walks forces us to log off and focus on our health and well-being. This helps us to get along better and enjoy each other even more. Honestly, I feel better about myself and proud of what my body can do, so I'm more happy and pleasant to be around.

"A few weeks ago we were walking and my husband had stepped behind me for a moment to allow another group to pass. He tapped me on the shoulder and said, *'Excuse me, ma'am, what's happened to my wife and where did this one come from? I like this energetic and active version of you!'*

"Although we have always been a close couple, after 17 years, walking together has given us a new level of time, focus, and energy for each other."

As Jennifer has experienced, walking with the people you love can have a profound, positive impact on your relationship. Much of what she and her husband experienced as a result of walking together is grounded in science and shared by the experiences of countless other couples. As a study from Brigham Young University showed, exercising together is linked to benefits for both spouses who "reported more positive marital events, fewer negative marital events, and higher marital satisfaction on days that they reported exercising together.

Don't Look Them In the Eyes: Walking with Your Teen

Dogs, wolves, chimpanzees, and other animal species perceive direct eye contact as aggressive, threatening behavior. Apparently, so do teens.

Early in my journey as the mother-of-a-teenager – around the time my firstborn turned 14 – I read an article that offered this valuable piece of advice: if you want your teenager to talk to you, treat them like a wild animal and don't look them in the eye. Crazy? Nope. Many parents will tell you that they have the best conversations with their teens while in the car. Or while walking. Bev Landgren experienced the power of shoulder-to-shoulder walking with her teenage son first-hand.

"Walking, we were side-by-side, not face-to-face, and he opened up a lot. Often, we walked during the evening or even after dark, and years later he told me that he felt a freedom in the dark and not looking me in the eye that he did not feel at other times."

She's not alone in experiencing the power of walking to connect with her teen.

"My daughter had a rough year," Rosalie Hull shared. "Really rough – wouldn't get out of bed rough. I started dragging her on walks. At first, she came kicking and screaming. Now she asks me every Friday night when we will be walking on Saturday. We start out talking about nothing, but usually about 15 minutes in, the real stuff comes out. And we walk until we have figured it out."

For Kara Cunny and her three daughters, "Do you want to take a walk?" has become a secret code for a private conversation. "Just yesterday, my 7th grader texted me from the bus on the way home asking if we could walk. On our walk, she told me about a friend who is threatening self harm and my daughter wanted to know how to get her help. We walked the block and I asked her if she felt better or wanted to go again. We ended up going around 3 times, chatting about all sorts of stuff. She likes walking and talking because she doesn't have to make eye contact and can channel nervous energy into steps."

None of this surprises Dr. David Krauss, a clinical psychologist who works with kids and teens and who offered to share his personal experience and professional insights. "I first discovered the power of walking with kids between college and graduate school," he explains. "I was working at an in-patient facility and was sometimes asked to help kids who were upset or being disruptive. I would take them outside to walk the grounds together and I noticed the way walking helped calm many kids and how I would sometimes hear things from them that I wouldn't hear inside." Years later – after graduate school and licensing and the launch of his own practice – Dr. Krauss rediscovered the power of walking sessions to foster engagement and cooperation. "For kids who tend to be argumentative," he explains, "walking in parallel and not looking them in the eye often helps," he explains.

Dr. Krauss has also seen benefits from walking with neuroatypical patients, particularly those with ADHD or autism. "For kids with ADHD, staying seated during therapy takes a lot of energy, but that's not an issue when we are walking," he explains. "And when you are talking face-to-face with a child with autism, he is often working to interpret your non-verbal clues and actively avoiding eye contact, both of which take a lot of cognitive energy – energy which they don't have to expend when we are walking side-by-side."

Last but not least, walking with his patients gives Dr. Krauss the chance to get their perspective on the world and share experiences. "Last week, I was walking with a patient and we noticed a hawk on a branch. We stood together for a moment just to watch and experience a real-life example of mindfulness, gratitude, and being present."

Besides the power of being side-by-side, are there other factors at play that make walking with your teen so powerful? I believe so.

First, they will be off their phones. Though I suppose it is possible for teens to walk and text – since it seems that they are able to do everything simultaneously with being plugged in and connected – chances are, especially with a gentle nudge from you (safety first), their phones will remain in their pockets.

And so will you. A 2019 survey commissioned by restaurant chain Red Robin revealed that 73% of kids wish that they had more quality time to connect with their parents. Yup, those teens who communicate their desire to be alone with rolled eyes, off-putting body language, and slammed doors might actually want more time with you. Walking together gives that to them … and to you.

Second, teens are moody – it just comes with the territory – and walking gives them all of the mood boosting power we've talked about. Give them just 10 minutes of walking, and watch those happy hormones start to flow.

Third, silence is more comfortable while you are walking. Embrace the silence, and resist any urge you have to force a conversation. If your teenager wants to listen to music and simply walk in compatible silence, let them. They will talk when they are ready.

And finally, you are teaching them, through your actions, the power of walking as a practice. You are modeling the importance of prioritizing movement, exercise, and restorative time.

All of this sounds great, right? But how in the world do you get a teenager who seems to have grown roots in their bedroom with their phone velcroed to their hand to lace up their sneakers and walk with you?

Like anything teenage-related, the answer is nuanced, inconsistent, and will likely take some time. Strive to invite rather than insist. Teenagers are wired to rebel, so forcing them to walk with you is unlikely to give you the shared experience you are hoping for. Second, accept that you might have to invite them to join you repeatedly and you are likely to get different answers – some days yes and some days no. Don't convey your disappointment, remember though they don't always let on about it, many teens are sensitive to feeling that they are disappointing you. Third, consider adding a destination that will entice them, take a walk to a favorite local coffee shop or head to the local animal shelter and walk dogs together. And, when they do join you, fight the urge to pepper them with questions. Leave any agenda at home and be willing to let the walk unfold as it is meant to.

Wanna' Go for a Walk and Fight? Walking and Conflict Resolution.

"Wanna' go for a walk and fight?" I asked Eric one Sunday morning. It was mid-pandemic, our business had hit several major speed bumps, and we had two teenagers living under our roof – one of whom was supposed to be away at college. Tempers were short and tensions were high.

Eric looked at me and sighed. "Okay," he said.

For several months, Eric and I had been heading out on walks together, usually two-and-a-half miles down a favorite dirt road. Invariably, I was the one who suggested it and often our conversations deteriorated into disagreements, arguments, or stormy silence. Eric had come to dub them "walk and fights." And yet, we kept taking those walks together.

They weren't always fun and we didn't miraculously resolve every issue or settle every disagreement during a single 40-minute walk. But even when the underlying issue lingered, we left the trail in better space than when disagreements bubbled up in the den and ended with us storming off to the opposite end of the house. Somehow, even when the conversations were difficult, we made more progress, had more peace, and seemed better able to see one another's point of view out on that trail.

This does not surprise Dr. Christine E. Webb, a professor in the Department of Human Evolutionary Biology at Harvard, and co-author of *"Stepping Forward Together: could walking facilitate interpersonal conflict resolution?"*

Dr. Webb's research study of walking and conflict resolution is a bit of a departure from her usual study of the behavior of primates. As we walked and talked, she shared what inspired her research. "I was intrigued by the differences in how humans versus other primates resolve conflict," she explained. "We humans like to talk all of the time and I've observed, through research and through my own experience, that with all that talking, we sometimes manage to create new conflicts rather than resolving the thing we were initially arguing about."

Yup, been there. More times than I can count. Eric and I will be disagreeing about one thing which will lead to some long, meandering conversation in which we end up digging in our heels and arguing about something else.

This dynamic is not unusual and can happen even when you don't care all that much about the underlying issue. What you care most about, even if you are unwilling to admit it, is being *right*. My guess, though I haven't ever asked them, is that primates care less about being right and more about resolving the conflict, making their troop member feel better, and moving on.

"I had also noticed how the words and phrases we use when we talk about conflict often reference movement – psychology literature is filled with it," Dr. Webb observed. "*Getting past it. Moving on. Putting it behind us.* And when we can't *move past it* we use phrases like *being stuck* or *at an impasse*."

Digging in our heels.

These observations, combined with her personal experience, led Dr. Webb and her colleagues to consider the question: Can walking help with conflict resolution?

Not surprisingly, their answer was yes.

"There are two major factors at play," she explains. "The first relates to the individual benefits of walking and the second to the interpersonal benefits."

The Individual Benefits

We've explored the many ways walking helps your mind work at its very best, several of which are helpful for conflict resolution: decreased stress, increased positive hormones, improved brain function, and all of the benefits that come from being in nature.

"Perhaps the most important of these for conflict resolution is the increase in creativity that comes with walking," Dr. Webb suggested. "The type of creativity that research shows is most strongly impacted by walking is 'divergent thinking' which, at its simplest, refers to our ability to see things in a different way. That type of thinking is instrumental to conflict resolution."

Ah, the ability to view a situation through someone else's eyes, to grasp their perspective – even if you disagree. Yup, that seems helpful for resolving conflict.

The Interpersonal Benefits

"Another key to the power of walking for conflict resolution is behavioral synchrony," Dr. Webb observes.

Behavioral synchrony has been linked to increased cooperation, compassion, and feelings of connection – all really helpful to two people who are trying to resolve a conflict.

We've discussed the physical synchronicity that often happens when people walk together, but, as Dr. Webb points out, there are other less obvious ways that we sync up when we walk together. "There are several implicit agreements we make when we walk with another person," Dr. Webb explains. "We agree on how fast we will walk, we agree when we turn. Our bodies are in implicit agreement and that helps to facilitate more constructive conversation."

Somehow, Eric and I rarely walk and fight these days. Rather, like Jennifer and her husband, we now use our walking time to connect, make plans, share ideas, or just walk side by side in companionable quiet. But occasionally, when there is an issue we need to address, I will invite him for a walk and fight. Usually, he says yes.

The Value of A Chat with a Stranger

We've explored the value of walking together to forge and deepen meaningful relationships, but what about those casual, impromptu exchanges with strangers? What can those encounters do for us?

It was a rainy Friday afternoon and I had been sent downtown to interview a witness. I don't recall the exact year, but it was long before you could summon a ride on your phone. Heck, it was before you could do anything on your phone other than use it as, well, a phone. I completed my meeting, packed my notes into my briefcase, took the elevator to the ground floor, and stepped out into a rainy New York City street.

There wasn't a taxi to be found as I stood on the corner with rain dripping off the edges of my umbrella and into my shoes. I contemplated walking the eight blocks to the nearest subway, but the thought of being squashed together with other rain-soaked New Yorkers in the bowels of the subway wasn't very appealing either. And just as I was getting close to giving up hope, a yellow taxi turned the corner and headed toward me, the illuminated rooftop light indicating that he was available. I stepped into the street and raised my arm in a gesture familiar to all New Yorkers. The cab pulled over and I opened the door at the exact same moment a man opened the door from the other side. "This is my cab," I barked, in a tone also familiar to all New Yorkers.

"No," the man said, "he stopped for me." And so began a brief scuffle, interrupted by the driver.

"I don't care who, but one of you, get in," he said.

"Wait, where are you going?" I asked.

"81st and Madison," the man said.

"I'm going to 46th and Fifth. Let's share it."

Soggy and dripping, we climbed into the back seat of the taxi and began the uptown crawl through late afternoon traffic. The man had two big bags which he placed on the floor between us. I peeked – they were filled with lingerie.

"Yours?" I asked with a smile. 'Cause we were sharing a cab, so now we were friends.

"Not exactly," he replied. "I'm a stylist for Victoria's Secret and I'm coming back from a shoot for our next catalog." Remember, this was years ago, back in the days when the Victoria's Secret catalog was the ultimate mashup of fashion magazine and soft porn. But oh, some of their bras were just beautiful. For the next 20 minutes, my new friend Kevin and I chatted. About his move to New York when he was 18, how he landed the job with Victoria's Secret more than a decade later, how the right undergarments can make a woman feel good, even when she is dressing just for herself, what it was like to be a 28-year-old lawyer working crazy hours and the boyfriend who didn't seem to adore her quite as much as she adored him. We were approaching my office at 46th and Fifth when Kevin looked at me and asked "34C?"

"Wow," I said, "you're good." And he reached into the shopping bag and pulled out three brightly colored, beautiful bras, the kind I never would have bought for myself. "Thank you," I said, giving him a warm hug before stepping back out into the cold rain.

I never saw him again and those three gorgeous bras are long, long gone. But even sitting here right now, that memory makes me smile. And it reminds me of the power of casual connections and conversations with strangers.

We place so much emphasis on the important relationships in our lives that we often discount the significance of impromptu exchanges with strangers. But aside from three gorgeous new bras, was there value in my conversation with a stranger in the back of a cab on that rainy Friday?

It was yet another rainy day when I had the chance to speak with Psychology Professor Dr. Gillian Sandstrom about this. For more than a decade, her research has focused on conversations with strangers, the kind of interactions you have with people you don't know and are unlikely to ever see again. She calls these interactions "little jewels" of human connection, which, her research shows, deliver four key benefits.

First, a conversation with a stranger benefits your mood: "people are generally in a better mood after they've talked with a stranger," she explained.

Second, these casual interactions provide a feeling of connection with other people, which is critical to our mental health and sense of wellbeing especially during times when we are feeling particularly disconnected or alone. "For instance, when you've recently moved to a new city, or been in lockdown during a global pandemic," Dr. Sandstrom said, reflecting on the value of conversations with strangers during the COVID pandemic. "For many people, taking walks was one the few things we were allowed to do. Those walks provided the opportunity to talk to people and for many those conversations were a lifesaver."

Third, talking with strangers fosters feelings of trust, not just in the person with whom you chat, but in people in general. "In one study," Dr. Sandstrom shared, "people reported a greater sense of trust in other people after just a single conversation with a stranger."

Finally, there's the opportunity to expand our horizons, shift our perspective and bring new ideas into our lives. "We learn a lot from other people and often more than we expect to, from complete strangers," she concluded.

And then there are the intangibles, the things that are difficult for a researcher to quantify, test, and study, but the benefits that add color, flavor, and fun to our lives.

"Recently," Dr. Sandstrom shared, "I was having kind of a rough day, so I thought I'd go for a longer-than-usual walk." By the end of her 5-mile walk, Dr. Sanstrom had met 12 dogs and been invited to join a book club by complete strangers. Well, they're not complete strangers anymore.

Walking to Build Community

Walking together can strengthen ties between individuals, but can walking transform neighborhoods and communities? Can walking together make the world a better place?

Yes. A resounding yes.

The Benefits of Walkable Communities

As I've mentioned, I've always been an early bird. I love to start my day before the rest of the world is fully awake. I love the preternatural quiet of the early morning and the chance to see the sun begin to peek over the horizon. I love the feeling that the coming day brings with it a world of possibilities.

When I was in my 20s, I lived and worked in New York City. I would wake around 6:00, pull on sweatpants, a sports bra, and a t-shirt and head out the door of my apartment building. Sometimes I would walk, sometimes I would jog. On my way back, I would stop at the coffee truck on the corner for my coveted morning coffee. I would chat with Harold, the elderly man who owned the coffee truck, usually about the weather. He would call me hon, short, of course, for honey, though I know he knew my name. I would take my coffee up to my apartment, shower, dry my hair, "put on my face," don a silk blouse, a lawyerly suit, and a comfortable pair of flats. Then back out the door for the half-mile walk to my office. Elevator to the 9th floor, greet Angel, my favorite receptionist, head down the hall to my office, slip off my flats, grab a pair of heels from the oversized bottom drawer of my desk, and get to work.

At the end of the day, the process would reverse: heels were exchanged for flats before the half-mile walk home, often stopping to chat with the doorman or the neighbors I encountered along the way.

If I wasn't traveling, I walked to and from work every single day. That's five miles a week, 50 weeks a year (assuming two weeks vacation). 250 miles each year.

Weekends often found me exploring different neighborhoods, walking two miles to Little Italy for the fresh pasta, all the way to the Upper West Side to visit my friend Julie, or to Union Square farmers market in search of the perfect tomato.

The first year I moved out of the city, I gained five pounds. Nothing changed... not my eating habits, not my morning jog. The only thing that changed was that 250 miles.

I realized how much I missed walking as the way to transition from home to work and back again. I missed the casual interactions with people and my morning conversation with Harold. I missed the sense of connection I felt with my neighborhood. And I was shocked by the impact on my body. Leaving one of the world's most walkable cities had an immediate impact on my health and my happiness.

The word "walkability" isn't actually a word, at least not according to the Oxford Dictionary, nor Merriam Webster. Nevertheless, the word has caught on in recent years with many arguing that walkable communities have a myriad of positive impacts on the lives of people who live in them.

William H. Whyte was a researcher, sociologist, and writer who, for much of his career, focused on questions of city planning and what it takes to create neighborhoods that offer the highest degree of connectedness and community. He was a pioneer in the study of how human beings interact in urban settings and how those insights can be used to improve our cities and our lives. Top of his list? Creating cities that encourage walking and interaction.

In 1969, Whyte was hired to help the New York City Planning Commission create a city plan, launching years of research into what makes a city vibrant, special, and happy. He spent 16 years meticulously observing the patterns of people in city spaces. How they walked, where they stopped, what they looked at, and where and when they chatted with others. His work helped to inform the creation of much urban planning and many public spaces.

Whyte called the city street "the river of life of the city, the place where we come together, the pathway to the center," and was one of the first to recognize the potential negative impact of what he called "undercrowding:"

> There is a rash of studies underway designed to uncover the bad consequences of overcrowding. This is all very well as far as it goes, but it only goes in one direction. What about undercrowding? The researchers would be a lot more objective if they paid as much attention to the possible effects on people of relative isolation and lack of propinquity.

Walking together has the power to help transform neighborhoods into communities. Why? How?

Picture this. You watch with curiosity as new neighbors move in across the street. How old are they? Do they have kids? Do they look nice? Perhaps you wander over to introduce yourself. Maybe you even bring them a pie. But it is unlikely that you will invite them over for dinner. For heaven's sake, you don't know them! Now imagine two different future scenarios.

In community number one, your neighborhood has no sidewalks and everyone gets into their cars in the morning, commutes to work, returns home, parks in their garages, and heads inside their home. Dinner, television, bed. Repeat.

In community number two, sidewalks, parks, and shops are within walking distance. After dinner, you often stroll through the neighborhood and Saturday mornings you walk to the local coffee shop. En route, you run into your new neighbor. "How are you finding the neighborhood?" you ask.

"Great," she responds, "though I've been trying to find a plumber; we are having an issue with the downstairs bathroom."

"Oh, I've got a great guy," you offer, pulling out your phone. "I'll text you his info, what's your number?"

A week later, you once again run into that new neighbor. "Hey, did you ever connect with the plumber?"

"Oh yes, he was great, thank you."

"Listen, I'm walking to Silbey's to get a cup of coffee. Wanna join?"

That is how neighbors begin to become friends.

These observations have been born out by researchers who have investigated what the invisible forces are that help residents of some communities feel more connected than residents of others.

In 2003, Dr. Kevin M. Leyden, then an Associate Professor from West Virginia University, sought to discover whether different types of neighborhoods led to different levels of social capital.

Social capital is generally defined as "the connections and inter-personal interactions that foster trust." Higher levels of social capital make people feel good and has been linked to increased political engagement, trust in others, and volunteerism. Dr. Leyden focused his study on residents of Galway, Ireland, a growing city that included a mix of neighborhood types including mixed-use, pedestrian-oriented of the sort built centuries before the automobile, and the contemporary "American-style" suburb.

He considered extensive survey data and concluded that people "living in walkable, mixed-use neighborhoods are more likely to know their neighbors, to participate politically, to trust others, and to be involved socially."

Forging new relationships takes time and repeated casual social interactions. Walkable neighborhoods provide lots of opportunities for those interactions. And, over time, as we'll learn momentarily from the experience of Shawn Dromgoole, walking together has the power to help dismantle barriers.

Shawn Dromgoole and The Walk Sound

In 1966, a young woman set out to buy a house with her widow's pension. She was pregnant, it was the South, and she was Black. But somehow she managed, securing a lovely home in a predominantly Black

Nashville neighborhood. There, she raised her daughter and – decades later – there her daughter raised her son Shawn Dromgoole. Shawn describes his childhood neighborhood as "a magical, almost fairytale-esque" place where everyone knew everyone, kids played outside, and if his home was out of chocolate ice cream, he'd just wander down the street to one of his aunt's freezers.

But over time, Shawn's neighborhood began to gentrify. Family and friends moved away and "the sense of community began to disappear," Shawn explains, "though you don't realize it as it is slowly trickling away." Shawn and his mother stayed, while the neighborhood became increasingly white.

Then in 2012 Trayvon Martin, an unarmed Black teenager returning home from a Skittles run, was shot and killed by a white man. A few years later, Ahmaud Arbery, an unarmed 25-year-old Black man, was shot while jogging in Georgia.

While these were hardly the only two unarmed Black men killed during that time, they struck Shawn hard: "I realized they could be me."

And then, in 2020, George Floyd's death at the hands of Minneapolis police officers was captured on video, igniting protests and a world-wide call for racial justice. Black Americans began to give voice to the challenges and fears they encounter daily.

"I put on a new pair of Nikes and had planned to go for a walk," Shawn says. "I wasn't consciously thinking about George Floyd, or Trayvon or anything else, but I literally couldn't go."

The next day, he tried again, but once again couldn't will himself off his front porch. "In retrospect," Shawn explains, "I realize that I was having a panic attack, though I didn't recognize it at the time." He called his mother who insisted he go and offered to walk with him. "She was not going to let me be afraid," he explains. The two walked and talked and laughed, but when they got home, "we began to feel angry," Shawn explains. Without intending to spark a movement, Shawn took to social media and posted this message:

> Yesterday, I wanted to walk around my neighborhood but the fear of not returning home to my family alive kept me on my front porch. Today, I wanted to walk again and I could not make it off the porch. Then I called my mother and she said she would walk with me.

Within minutes, neighbors replied, offering to walk with Shawn. And the next day, they did. "100 people showed up to walk with me." The media got hold of the story and the next week, Shawn found 300 people gathered in his front yard for a community walk. As they walked, other neighbors joined from their front porches. "People who lived two houses from one another met for the first time and walked and talked."

Shawn's neighbors continue to walk. Friendships have been created and the sense of community has begun to return to the neighborhood. And Shawn has taken his mission on the road with the creation of the not-for-profit *We Walk with Shawn*, sharing his story and transforming neighborhoods into communities through the power of walking together.

"My favorite thing about the walks is what I call The Walk Sound – the chatter I hear behind me when we are walking. That's the sound of new relationships growing and communities being built."

A Walking School Bus

It's the stuff of many movies and countless TV shows. Elementary school student, let's call her Suzy, gets up, gets dressed, grabs her lunch from the kitchen counter, kisses her mom goodbye, hoists her backpack to her shoulder, and walks to school. Along the way she stops to pick up her friend "Beth" who lives down the block. "Alice" joins as they get closer to school, while a similar group of three boys follows a bit behind. They talk about the day to come, how mean their math teacher is, and maybe about the three boys trailing behind them. At the end of the day, the process reverses. The conversation again turns to the mean math teacher, or the silly thing someone said during Spanish class. When they get to Alice's house, they head in together to do homework, eat cookies, and continue their conversation. For decades, this scenario played out in neighborhoods across the country.

Now picture this: Suzy waits for the bus, earbuds in place. She gets on the bus where, in every row, kids' eyes are downcast, staring at their phones. Beth gets on the bus, smiles at Suzy, but, observing the bus culture, remains quiet, sits down and opens the latest app. Alice, who lives just one block from school, walks there by herself, listening to a podcast. At the end of the day, the process is reversed, with the girls lost in their own private worlds, decamping to their own homes. Perhaps they will connect later on social media.

Juliet Starrett found a solution. She is the founder of StandUp Kids – a not-for-profit on a mission to educate parents and teachers about the negative effects of too much sitting – and the co-author with her husband Kelly of *Built to Move*. The importance of movement is core to the Starrett family's DNA, so it comes as no surprise that their solution to the stress of morning drop-off involved walking.

"Kelly and I had this realization that our mornings had become un-pleasant and unnecessarily stressful – sitting in traffic, waiting in the drop-off line. We live a mile from school and one day we said, 'Let's just walk our daughter to school.' So that's what we did. Kelly and I would walk Caroline to school, drop her off, and walk home together. Immediately, our mornings became more peaceful. At the time, I was doing research for StandUp Kids and the concept of a 'Walking School Bus' crossed my radar. We had already experienced how nice it was to walk our daughter to school and I thought there must be other parents in our neighborhood who might embrace this idea."

Juliet shared the plan at back-to-school night. "I explained that every day, rain or shine, we would meet at a specific corner at 7:50 and walk the kids to school. I started with a few friends and set up a schedule so that we knew there would be at least one parent there every day," and the neighborhood's Walking School Bus was born.

"Based on all of the research I was doing about the negative impact of too much sitting, I knew the Walking School Bus would be good for the children, and pretty quickly I heard from teachers who agreed. They would say things like 'the kids on the Walking School Bus get all of their wiggles out' and arrive at school awake and ready to learn.'"

But what Juliet didn't anticipate was the impact it would have on the parents and the community. "Each day, the assigned parent was there, but often there would be five, six, or even ten other parents who would walk too." Juliet says. "No one was on their phone and it gave the parents the opportunity to really get to know one another." As the months went by, Juliet says, "lifelong friendships were created."

A Walking Classroom

Christi Hartley teaches 5th grade. Twice a week for the past six years, she and her students grab audio players and head outside to walk a mile while listening to a special lesson. "Typically, the lessons include a health lesson – like what happens in your brain while you walk, or what kinds of foods are best to eat before you walk – followed by a more traditional lesson in language arts or social studies or science," she explains. "It has been phenomenal for my students," she says.

Christi is one of 6,800 teachers who participate in The Walking Classroom, a program created more than a decade ago by 5th grade teacher Laura Fenn. "I used to play kickball with my students every Friday afternoon. One day, the principal told me I couldn't do that anymore because it was taking away from instructional time," Laura explained when we spoke. But she had seen the positive impact of physical activity and wasn't willing to give up on finding a way to get her students the activity she knew they needed. The solution came to her weeks later while she was, not surprisingly, on a walk.

"I had come home from work in a terrible mood after a really, really bad day. I didn't want to talk to anyone, so I went for a walk and listened to a podcast. While I was walking, my mood improved, I was getting some desperately needed fresh air and exercise, and I was learning something. I thought, '*My students could do this.*' I went home and began recording a few lessons I would have taught to my students while they were sitting in the classroom. I bought several cheap mp3 players and asked my principal if I could take my students to the forbidden world of the *outside*. I explained that it was still *me* teaching, but the kids were going to listen to the lesson while we walked." To Laura's surprise, the principal agreed.

Laura's goal had been simply to get the students outside for some fresh air and exercise. "I didn't expect them to learn much from my audio lessons, but I had to use that "teach-y" part to convince my principal that I wasn't sacrificing instructional time. I knew the students would be primed for learning after they got some fresh air and exercise, but I honestly didn't think they'd retain much of what they listened to while we were out."

What happened surprised her. "Of course, they loved getting outside, but I was shocked by how much they retained. And it turned out that my struggling readers, my ADHD kids, my kids with autism, dyslexia, and behavioral issues were the best listeners and could share nearly word-for-word what they had learned. It was amazing."

Laura continued her homemade program for two years before leaving the classroom to stay home with her own kids. "While I was home, I developed the program more thoroughly, hired teachers to create additional lesson plans, and recorded them." Ten years later, The Walking Classroom is going strong and is being used to educate more than 700,000 kids across the country.

"The Walking Classroom has been phenomenal for my students," says Christi Hartley. "They absorb ten-fold the information and I've seen them get stronger and fitter throughout the year." She recalled a particular student the first year she introduced The Walking Classroom to her class. "In 5th grade, she was already 5' 9" and over 200 pounds. When we started the program, she couldn't walk the entire mile, so she would walk what she could and then sit down on a bench to listen to the rest of the lesson and rejoin the group at the end. By the end of the year, she was jogging some of that mile and passed every assessment without any help."

And today?

"She still texts me from time to time to share how she's doing and to tell me that she is keeping up with both her physical activity and her education."

The Power of Walking Groups

A few years ago, I decided to create a local walking group. As a busy business owner, mom of two kids and one dog, and all of the responsibilities that come with all of these things, I felt that my social circle had been shrinking – right along with my patience. I had gained a few pounds and missed the kinds of long meandering conversations experienced while walking. I sent an email to a dozen friends. "Let's create a walking group," I shouted with a bunch of exclamation points. *"Each Thursday morning at 8:00 a.m., anyone who is free, let's meet at the top of Barcelona Neck. We'll do the two-mile dirt road, though anyone who wants to stay for 'bonus miles' and do another two, that will work too. Well-behaved dogs welcome! Let's do this!"*

Sounds good, right? I committed to being there each Thursday morning and I assumed that some of my friends would just show up.

It was a total flop. Each week, when I sent out the reminder email, I would receive a half-dozen replies which mostly included some version of "sorry, too busy." After six weeks, I gave up.

Apparently, I was right and I was wrong.

I was right about the power of a walking group to give me the movement, the connection, and the conversations I was craving. But I wasn't quite right about how to get one going, so I consulted Dr. Sarah Hanson of the University of East Anglia.

In 2015, Dr. Hanson set out to ascertain whether or not the prescription to join a walking group should be a tool in the arsenal of medical professionals. "At the time," she explained when we spoke, "health professionals would sometimes recommend that patients join a walking group, but it wasn't well researched. I wanted to do the research so that practitioners could confidently prescribe walking."

After evaluating more than 5,000 walking studies, Dr. Hanson and her team identified tremendous benefits to being part of a walking group and concluded that "walking groups are effective and safe with good adherence and wide-ranging health benefits. They could be a promising intervention as an adjunct to other healthcare or as a proactive health-promoting activity."

Their research confirmed what others had consistently demonstrated: Walking has tremendous benefits to many health measures including blood pressure, heart rate, body fat, BMI, cholesterol, depression, and quality of life, all with a high level of adherence and a low risk of serious adverse effects. "Not to overstate it," Dr. Hanson said, "but walking is a wonder drug."

That's all well and good – but like any exercise-based prescription, a walking program only works if people do it. And that was the key discovery. "When people join a walking group, they tend to stick with it," she explained.

Why? Dr. Hanson and her colleagues identified three key reasons why being part of a walking group encourages consistency.

First is the sense of social adherence. "If you say 'I'll see you next week' you've made a social commitment and you are far more likely to show up," she explained.

Second, being part of a walking group creates social connectedness and social support which are critical to well-being. Dr. Hanson told me about one woman she had interviewed who said that if it weren't for her walking group, she wouldn't see or interact with anyone else during the entire week.

Last, but not least, people enjoy it – "people will only stick with doing something that they enjoy," and the research shows that people enjoy walking with others.

Not only do people keep turning up, but it turns out they do more during their walks. "We discovered that people walked further and faster when they walked with a group," Dr. Hanson concluded.

So what in the world did I do wrong when I tried to create my Thursday morning walking group? According to Dr. Hanson, a few things.

First, I launched my walking group in the summer, which seemed to make sense to me – the weather was great, kids were out of school, schedules tended to be lighter. But nope – according to her research, it's not great to launch a walking group in the summer because people's schedules tend to be varied and busy.

Second, perhaps I started with too large a group so that the dozen people I invited didn't feel like they were part of something and were missing out on any sense of social responsibility to one another.

Finally, perhaps I didn't give it long enough to catch on and grow. Or maybe a few people needed to get there at least one time to discover the social support that they would get from one another.

Maybe I need to try again.

***

Over the past two decades, I have taken countless walks with count-less people. With my husband, my kids, and my friends. Couples walks where, seemingly invariably and despite our best efforts, midway through the walk, the women and the men separate into smaller gender-specific groups with the dogs running back and forth between us. Walks with acquaintances who later become friends and with those who didn't.

I can't contemplate the thousands of conversations shared and the confidences exchanged on those walks. They have been a balm to virtually every difficult thing I have navigated over the past two decades and have also brought fun, laughter, endorphins, serotonin, dopamine and oxytocin. They have reduced my stress and increased my happiness, strengthened my bones and burned more calories than I could possibly calculate. On my calendar today is a 10:15 walk with my neighbor Dora and a 6:30 walk with my cousin Nina. I'm looking forward to them both.

Sometimes people tell me, "I wish I had someone to walk with" or "I wish I had time to walk." And it is not just people with sedentary jobs, or who don't know the importance of physical activity. At a fitness-industry cocktail party, I had a conversation with the president of a multi-million-dollar fitness company. "I really should walk more," she said. "There are so many days I never get up from my desk, and I know that's not good." You never get up from your desk? Seriously, you run a fitness company. I didn't say that. But I thought it.

Okay, so you wish you walked more and you wish you had friends to walk with. I get it. And I promise you, you can have that.

First, the time issue. Find your time confetti. Start by finding five minutes here or then ten minutes there. Start small. Walk around the building while you are at work or around the block before the kids get up. Put a 20-minute walk on your calendar on Friday afternoons as a way to end your work week. Walk after dinner (even if you don't feel like it). Add an extra 10 minutes to your dog's evening walk.

Second, the friends-to-walk-with issue. Remember the woman I mentioned early on who shared that she felt like she didn't have a single close friend in the world? She is not alone in feeling that way. There are millions of people right this moment, this very second, who feel lonely and wish they had a walking companion. You could be that companion.

You are going to have to put yourself out there, at least a little bit. Go first. Extend the invitation.

"But wait," you're saying, "I don't have anyone to invite." But are you sure? Is there a neighbor you greet when you see them? A cousin who lives a few miles away? Someone you work with and with whom you find yourself chatting just a few minutes longer than just a cordial hello? A person you see at church or synagogue or your mosque, community house, place of worship, AA meeting or your daughter's gymnastics practice?

Go ahead. Go first. Anything along the lines of "Hey, I've been trying to get a little more exercise these days and was thinking it might be nice to take a walk [after services, during lunch, in the mornings, while the kids are in class] any interest in joining me?"

Scary, right? And yup, they might say no.

But, as we tell our kids, you don't ask, you don't get.

So go ahead. Ask. Invite. Go first. Take the risk. And – and this part is really, really important – if they say no ... ask someone else. Take the initiative. Build your walking tribe.

Go.

Conclusion

When You Need it Most, You Will Feel Like it Least

Over the past many hours together, we've explored the power of a regular walking practice to reduce your risk of developing a myriad of diseases, reverse others, and slow the progress of even more. We've talked about how we can walk ourselves happier, combat depression, and discover awe. We have learned that walking can help us sleep better and improve our relationships. I've shared stories of people who have walked their way to better and reams of research establishing – beyond doubt – that a regular walking practice can add years to your life and help you live each of those years healthier and happier.

And so much more.

So you would think that every one of us would burst out of bed in the morning, ready to take on a two, three, or five-mile walk and close out our days with a neighborhood stroll. You would assume that walking would be like brushing our teeth – a habit that we know is good for us, that makes us feel better, and that we simply do every day.

You'd be wrong. Instead, we long for the comfort of our comforters and the safety of our homes. We would rather sit on the couch than brave the elements. And this urge to stay home, to move less and eat more becomes even more pronounced the less you move. When your back aches or your knees feel creaky. When a good night sleep has eluded you and your energy is low. When a poor diet has sapped your vitality and added a few pounds – or more than a few – to your midsection. When you feel stressed or anxious or when you are confronting a work deadline you are afraid you won't meet. When you are experiencing grief or loss or fear or frustration.

At times like those, few think: "I'm going to put all this aside and go for a walk."

Because – and here's the rub – ***when you need it most, you will feel like it least.***

When we don't have a regular walking practice, getting started can be very difficult. Who has the time to add one more thing to your plate? And even when we have managed to create a walking habit, when our routine gets interrupted – as it inevitably will – it becomes very difficult to get going again.

Every one, no matter the level of activity in their life, has experienced this. When you are in a groove, in a habit, in a pattern, in a routine of regular movement, it seems relatively easy to keep going. But once life, or weather, or illness, or injury, or work, or family, or grief, or a new job, new baby, new puppy, fresh wave of depression, or … whatever … causes a break in that habit or disruption to that routine, getting going again becomes far, far more difficult.

Because when you need it most, you will feel like it least.

Researchers from the University of British Columbia employed brain scans to try to better understand what they called the "exercise paradox" – we know we should be more physically active, but clearly knowledge is not enough. In fact, despite the fact that "most individuals are now aware of the positive effects of regular physical activity and have the intention to exercise, from 2010 to 2016, the number of *in*active adults increased by 5% worldwide. Now, more than 1 in 4 adults fail to get sufficient activity," explains Professor Matthieu Boisgontier of the University of Ottawa.

Clearly, knowledge and intention are not enough to get us moving. Why? Why isn't it enough to know that we should? Shouldn't we *want* to do things that will make us stronger, healthier, and happier?

The paradox is caused by the intersection of two conflicting aspects of our evolutionary wiring: our need to move versus our need to conserve energy.

Once again, it goes back to our ancient ancestors who lived in caves and foraged for food. Life was hard, food was often scarce and the goal was to conserve as much energy as possible. By necessity, they moved plenty. Long arduous walks were part of life: by some estimates, they walked between four and nine miles each day. As a result, when they weren't forced to expend energy, when they weren't compelled to confront the dangers that lurked outside their caves, they wisely stayed put. As Professor Boisgontier explains, human beings have adapted to conserve energy so as to postpone "energy exhaustion" thereby increasing the odds of survival. In short, over the millennia, our bodies have learned it is better not to expend energy when we don't have to.

That ancient wiring is still within you. It tells your body to stay inside, avoid the elements, conserve energy, and avoid risk. It is the voice insisting that you are better off staying on the couch.

You need to be stronger than the voice of your ancient ancestors. You need to do the things that will contribute to the quality of your life, the things that will boost your mood, help your brain and improve your health and longevity, even when you don't feel like it. Especially when you don't feel like it.

How do you overcome that inertia? How do you get off the couch despite thousands of years of evolution telling you to stay put? Professor Boisgontier has some advice.

"To overcome that inertia, we need to develop habits related to physical activity and exercise. We need to help our brains automatically make choices associated with higher energy expenditure and thus make self-control unnecessary. When it comes to exercise, especially in the beginning, we need to learn that just showing up is success and focus on attendance, not effort. And we need to surround our workouts with positivity to increase the likelihood that our brain associates physical activity with positive feelings."

This is where the industrial fitness complex has failed us. They have told us, over and over and over again, that fitness and wellness look a certain way. They have admonished us that without pain there is no gain. They have lured us into believing that if our physical activity effort doesn't reach a certain threshold we just shouldn't bother. They have convinced us that exercise is punishment for a piece of pie, and that we can somehow hate ourselves healthy.

All of this is wrong. Every step counts, every mile matters, and trying is succeeding. What works for her might not work for you, and that is okay. Striving to fit into some ideal, or into your "skinny jeans," is neither a recipe for vitality nor happiness.

There is no end goal. There is just this journey and on this journey, every step counts and every mile matters.

He's Still My Dad

"Let's take a walk," my dad suggested. As I often am in my visits, I was sitting at the kitchen table in their home in Florida, working. I had come down for a visit after my parents received their COVID vaccines. I hadn't seen them in many, many months and they had not been easy months. Two falls had landed my dad in rehab where he experienced terrible loneliness and depression. He recovered and returned home. A few months later, he and my mother received their COVID vaccines, and here I was.

"Okay," I said, closing my computer, "let's go."

My dad grabbed the cane that he doesn't need except on those occasions when he does and I grabbed my sunglasses. We walked out the front door into the bright Florida sunshine.

My dad is 92. Other than the falls and a doctor who keeps a close eye on his kidneys, he's okay. He's still 100% my dad. He prepares his own breakfast and, though my mother does most of the cooking, he washes every dish. When I call, he instantly recognizes my voice and starts every conversation with the same "*hey babe*" greeting I have heard all of my life. He knows me better than just about anyone and still shines his love, his light and his insights on everyone he meets. Okay, so his hearing isn't perfect, he sometimes loses the thread of a television show, and has come to appreciate an afternoon nap.

"Daddy," I asked, "what do you attribute your longevity to?" I knew the answer, but I wanted to hear it from him, because I wanted to share it with you, in his words.

"Exercise," he replied. "Plain and simple. The older I get the more convinced I am that exercise is the key."

Did I mention that my dad is 92?

I have walked thousands of hours with my parents. I have walked thousands of hours with my husband, with my friends, and by myself. Though I have done – and continue to do – many other forms of exercise throughout my life, walking has been the one constant. As I've said, I have shaken off more stress, created more ideas, processed more difficult things, and yes, burned more calories walking than through any other habit or practice.

When I first set out to write a book about the transformative power of a regular walking practice, I worried that I would not have enough to talk about. I know through my own experience and bottomless research that walking is transformative. But could I share the data in a way that was interesting? Would other people be willing to tell me their stories honestly? Most importantly, could I find a way to convey it all in a way that would inspire and motivate others?

I wasn't sure.

Nevertheless, I set out on this journey to synthesize everything I know from my own experience, from the stories of others, and from thousands of hours of research in hopes of inspiring as many people as possible to embrace the transformative power of a regular walking practice.

It turns out, there was more than enough.

Finally, A Tale of September 11 and Knowing You Can, If You Had To

The sky was an exceptionally bright, infinite blue, the air was clear, and the temperature was that sweet spot where just a light jacket will do. Sunglasses were a must. All in all, it was a spectacular September day.

I was on a bus for the 90-mile ride from my home in Southampton to midtown Manhattan where I was scheduled to take a deposition, ironically of a man who worked for the department of defense, at 1:00. Earlier that morning, I had dropped my ten-month-old son at daycare, put on my favorite navy blue suit, and gathered my notes. We were about 10 minutes from the Queens Midtown Tunnel, a mile-long tunnel that runs under the East River and connects Long Island to Manhattan, when dozens of cellphones began to ring at just about the same moment.

It was September 11, 2001. Moments before, the first plane had struck Tower One of the World Trade Center, a building my great uncle had helped to engineer. When I was a kid, my mother used a piece of marble from the lobby as a cheese board – my uncle had rescued it from the scrap heap and given it to her as a gift. As a result, I'd always felt a connection to the Twin Towers and remember running my hands over the marble in the lobby every time I visited the two iconic buildings.

The bus inched slowly toward the mouth of the tunnel. For the moment, it was just a tragic plane crash. In the distance, we could see smoke pouring from the side of one of the world's tallest buildings. The tollbooth was about a dozen cars away when the second plane hit. It was no longer just a tragic plane crash, it was something more.

For several minutes that felt like an eternity, the bus was immobile: do we press forward into the city or turn and head back to Southampton? Every passenger who could get a call through was on their phone while the driver spoke anxiously via radio with dispatch. In those moments, I began to calculate. 90 miles stood between me and my infant son. If I push, I walk four miles an hour, so I could walk home in just over 22 hours. But wait, it was only 16 miles between me and the home of my Aunt Wendy and Uncle Norman. I could walk to their house in four or five hours, borrow a car, and be home before 6:00.

"We are turning around," the driver said, "and heading back to Southampton." The bus erupted. Some passengers, myself included, were relieved – our families were back where we had left them. Others were besides themselves because their loved ones were on the other side of that tunnel. "Let me out," one man insisted. "Now. Let me out. I'll walk," he insisted. A chorus of "yes, let me out too," rang out and the driver stopped, opened the door, and about thirty people got off the bus, uncertain and confused, but determined to cross the last miles into Manhattan on foot.

There is power in knowing that your two feet can enable you to cross tremendous distances. If they had to.

During the vast majority of our time on this planet, human beings were nomadic, moving from place to place in search of better: better weather, better soil, better hunting, better neighbors. For millennia, we made those journeys on foot. That spirit continues to reside within every one of us, buried beneath the perceived convenience of hopping in our car and driving to the coffee shop.

A regular walking practice reconnects us with an essential element of our nature. It empowers us by reminding us that we have the ability to get from here to there under our own power.

No one should ever have to contemplate fleeing a terrorist attack on foot to get to their infant son. But trust me, it is incredibly empowering to know that you could.

References

Introduction

1. 'This is Why Eating Healthy Is Hard (Time-Traveling Dietitian)', Funny or Die. <https://www.youtube.com/watch?v=5Ua-WVg1SsA>.

2. 'Adult Obesity Facts,' Centers for Disease Control and Prevention, May 17, 2022 <https://www.cdc.gov/obesity/data/adult.html>.

3. 'Major Depression: The Impact on Overall Health'. Blue Cross Blue Shield Report, May 10, 2018. <https://www.bcbs.com/the-health-of-america/reports/major-depression-the-impact-overall-health>.

Walking Makes Your Brain More Plastic (and that's a good thing)

4. Morais VAC, Tourino MFDS, Almeida ACS, Albuquerque TBD, Linhares RC, Christo PP, Martinelli PM, Scalzo PL. 'A single session of moderate intensity walking increases brain-derived neurotrophic factor (BDNF) in the chronic post-stroke patients'. Top Stroke Rehabil. 2018 Jan;25(1): 1-5. doi: 10.1080/10749357.2017.1373500. Epub 2017 Oct 27. PMID: 29078742.

5. Erickson, K. I., Voss, M. W., Prakash, R. S., Basak, C., Szabo, A., Chaddock, L., Kim, J. S., Heo, S., Alves, H., White, S. M., Wojcicki, T. R., Mailey, E., Vieira, V. J., Martin, S. A., Pence, B. D., Woods, J. A., McAuley, E., & Kramer, A. F. (2011). 'Exercise training increases size of hippocampus and improves memory'. Proceedings of the National Academy of Sciences, 108(7), 3017-3022. <https://doi.org/10.1073/pnas.1015950108>.

Stronger Scaffolding: Walking Builds More Efficient White Matter

6. Mendez Colmenares A, Voss MW, Fanning J, Salerno EA, Gothe NP, Thomas ML, McAuley E, Kramer AF, Burzynska AZ. 'White matter plasticity in healthy older adults: The effects of aerobic exercise'. Neuroimage. 2021 Oct 1; 239:118305. doi: 10.1016/j.neuroimage.2021.118305. Epub 2021 Jun 24. PMID: 34174392.

I Wonder Where that Trail Goes: Walking and Executive Function

7. Byun, K., Hyodo, K., Suwabe, K., Ochi, G., Sakairi, Y., Kato, M., Dan, I., & Soya, H. (2014). 'Positive effect of acute mild exercise on executive

function via arousal-related prefrontal activations: An fNIRS study'. NeuroImage, 98, 336-345. <https://doi.org/10.1016/j.neuroimage. 2014.04.067>.

What Can You Do With a Pillow: Walking and Creativity

8. Oppezzo M, Schwartz DL. 'Give your ideas some legs: the positive effect of walking on creative thinking.' J Exp Psychol Learn Mem Cogn. 2014 Jul;40(4):1142-52. doi: 10.1037/a0036577. Epub 2014 Apr 21. PMID: 24749966. <https://www.apa.org/pubs/journals/releases/xlm-a0036577.pdf>.

9. Rominger, C., Fink, A., Weber, B., Papousek, I., & Schwerdtfeger, A. R. (2020). 'Everyday bodily movement is associated with creativity independently from active positive affect: A Bayesian mediation analysis approach'. Scientific Reports, 10(1), 1-9. <https://doi.org/10.1038/s41598-020-68632-9>.

Getting Unstuck: Walking and Problem Solving

10. Cal Newport, 2016, Deep Work, Grand Central Publishing.

Squirrel: Walking and Improved Focus

11. Reviews.org surveyed 1,000 Americans aged 18 and above <https://www.reviews.org/mobile/cell-phone-addiction/>.

12. Basso JC, Suzuki WA. 'The Effects of Acute Exercise on Mood, Cognition, Neurophysiology, and Neurochemical Pathways: A Review'. Brain Plast. 2017 Mar 28;2(2):127-152. doi: 10.3233/BPL-160040. PMID: 29765853; PMCID: PMC5928534.

I Could Use a Few More Points: Walking and IQ

13. Aberg MA, Pedersen NL, Torén K, Svartengren M, Bäckstrand B, Johnsson T, Cooper-Kuhn CM, Aberg ND, Nilsson M, Kuhn HG. 'Cardiovascular fitness is associated with cognition in young adulthood'. Proc Natl Acad Sci U S A. 2009 Dec 8;106(49):20906-11. doi: 10.1073/pnas.0905307106. Epub 2009 Nov 30. PMID: 19948959; PMCID: PMC2785721.

Now, Where Did I Leave My Keys? Walking Improves Memory.

14. Suwabe, K., Byun, K., Hyodo, K., Reagh, Z. M., Roberts, J. M., Matsushita, A., Saotome, K., Ochi, G., Fukuie, T., Suzuki, K., Sankai, Y., Yassa, M. A., & Soya, H. (2018). 'Rapid stimulation of human dentate gyrus function with acute mild exercise'. Proceedings of the National Academy of Sciences, 115(41), 10487-10492. https://doi.org/10.1073/pnas.1805668115 <https://www.pnas.org/content/115/41/10487>.

15. Aleksandar Aksentijevicab, Kaz R.Brandta, EliasTsakanikosa, Michael J.A.Thorpe, 'It takes me back: The mnemonic time-travel effect', Cognition, Volume 182, January 2019, Pages 242-250.

My Dad is Still My Dad: Walking, Dementia, and Alzheimers

16. Etgen T, Sander D, Huntgeburth U, Poppert H, Förstl H, Bickel H. 'Physical Activity and Incident Cognitive Impairment in Elderly Persons: The INVADE Study.' Arch Intern Med. 2010;170(2):186–193. doi:10.1001/archinternmed.2009.498.

17. Nagamatsu LS, Chan A, Davis JC, Beattie BL, Graf P, Voss MW, Sharma D, Liu-Ambrose T. 'Physical activity improves verbal and spatial memory in older adults with probable mild cognitive impairment: a 6-month randomized controlled trial.' J Aging Res. 2013;2013:861893. doi: 10.1155/2013/861893. Epub 2013 Feb 24. PMID: 23509628; PMCID: PMC3595715.

Perhaps it is the Power of our Default Mode Network

18. Ferris Jabr, 'Why Walking Helps Us Think,' The New Yorker, September 3, 2014.

Perhaps it is the Boost in Brain-Derived Neurotrophic Factor (BDNF)

19. Ribeiro D, Petrigna L, Pereira FC, Muscella A, Bianco A, Tavares P. 'The Impact of Physical Exercise on the Circulating Levels of BDNF and NT 4/5: A Review'. Int J Mol Sci. 2021 Aug 16;22(16):8814. doi: 10.3390/ijms22168814. PMID: 34445512; PMCID: PMC8396229.

20. Morais VAC, Tourino MFDS, Almeida ACS, Albuquerque TBD, Linhares RC, Christo PP, Martinelli PM, Scalzo PL. 'A single session of moderate intensity walking increases brain-derived neurotrophic factor (BDNF) in the chronic post-stroke patients.' Top Stroke Rehabil. 2018 Jan;25(1): 1-5. doi: 10.1080/10749357.2017.1373500. Epub 2017 Oct 27. PMID: 29078742.

Fire Up the Positive Hormones

21. Basso JC, Suzuki WA. 'The Effects of Acute Exercise on Mood, Cognition, Neurophysiology, and Neurochemical Pathways: A Review.' Brain Plast. 2017 Mar 28;2(2):127-152. doi: 10.3233/BPL-160040. PMID: 29765853; PMCID: PMC5928534.

22. Jurado-Fasoli L, Di X, Sanchez-Delgado G, Yang W, Osuna-Prieto FJ, Ortiz-Alvarez L, Krekels E, Harms AC, Hankemeier T, Schönke M, Aguilera CM, Llamas-Elvira JM, Kohler I, Rensen PCN, Ruiz JR, Martinez-Tellez B. 'Acute and long-term exercise differently modulate plasma levels of oxylipins, endocannabinoids, and their analogues in young sedentary adults.' eBioMedicine, October 27, 2022, <https://doi.org/10.1016/j.ebiom.2022.104313>.

23. Kobayashi H, Song C, Ikei H, Park BJ, Kagawa T, Miyazaki Y. 'Combined Effect of Walking and Forest Environment on Salivary Cortisol Concentration.' Front Public Health. 2019 Dec 12;7:376. doi: 10.3389/fpubh.2019.00376. PMID: 31921741; PMCID: PMC6920124.

Walking Helps Combat Depression and Anxiety

24. If you believe you might be suffering from depression, there is help available. If you are uncertain where to start, the US Department of Health and Human Services has a free, confidential helpline that can provide you with information and connect you with local treatment facilities, support groups, and community organizations. They can be reached 24/7 at 1-800-662-4357 (help). The National Suicide Prevention Hotline is 800-273-8255.

25. P. C. Dinas; Y. Koutedakis; A. D. Flouris (2011). 'Effects of exercise and physical activity on depression'. Irish Journal of Medical Science (1971-), 180(2), 319–325. doi:10.1007/s11845-010-0633-9 .

26. Pearce M, Garcia L, Abbas A, et al. 'Association Between Physical Activity and Risk of Depression: A Systematic Review and Meta-analysis.' JAMA Psychiatry. 2022;79(6):550–559. doi:10.1001/jamapsychiatry.2022.0609.

27. Anxiety and Depression Association of America, 'Exercise for Stress and Anxiety', <https://adaa.org/living-with-anxiety/managing-anxiety/exercise-stress-and-anxiety>.

Rumination and Walking

28. Nejad AB, Fossati P, Lemogne C. 'Self-referential processing, rumination, and cortical midline structures in major depression.' Front Hum Neurosci. 2013 Oct 10;7:666. doi: 10.3389/fnhum.2013.00666. PMID: 24124416; PMCID: PMC3794427; Allaert J, De Raedt R, van der Veen FM, Baeken C, Vanderhasselt MA. Prefrontal tDCS attenuates counterfactual thinking in female individuals prone to self-critical rumination. Sci Rep. 2021 Jun 2;11(1):11601. doi: 10.1038/s41598-021-90677-7. PMID: 34078934; PMCID: PMC8172930.

29. Brand S, Colledge F, Ludyga S, Emmenegger R, Kalak N, Sadeghi Bahmani D, Holsboer-Trachsler E, Pühse U, Gerber M. 'Acute Bouts of Exercising Improved Mood, Rumination and Social Interaction in Inpatients With Mental Disorders'. Front Psychol. 2018 Mar 13;9:249. doi: 10.3389/fpsyg.2018.00249. PMID: 29593592; PMCID: PMC5859016.

30. Bratman, G. N., Hamilton, J. P., Hahn, K. S., Daily, G. C., & Gross, J. J. (2015). 'Nature experience reduces rumination and subgenual prefrontal cortex activation'. Proceedings of the National Academy of Sciences, 112(28), 8567-8572. <https://doi.org/10.1073/pnas.1510459112>.

Walking Can Help You Process Difficult Things

31. Williams J, Shorter GW, Howlett N, Zakrzewski-Fruer J, Chater AM. 'Can Physical Activity Support Grief Outcomes in Individuals Who Have Been Bereaved? A Systematic Review'. Sports Med Open. 2021 Apr 8;7(1):26. doi: 10.1186/s40798-021-00311-z. PMID: 33830368; PMCID: PMC8028581.

Walking Helps You Discover Awe

32. Bryan E. Robinson Ph.D., 'What Are "Awe Walks?" And why is a new study praising them?', Psychology Today Blog, November 3, 2020 <https://www.psychologytoday.com/us/blog/the-right-mindset/202011/what-are-awe-walks>.

33. Sturm, V. E., Datta, S., Roy, A. R. K., Sible, I. J., Kosik, E. L., Veziris, C. R., Chow, T. E., Morris, N. A., Neuhaus, J., Kramer, J. H., Miller, B. L., Holley, S. R., & Keltner, D. (2020, September 21). 'Big Smile, Small Self: Awe Walks Promote Prosocial Positive Emotions in Older Adults.' Emotion. Advance online publication. <http://dx.doi.org/10.1037/emo0000876>.

Better Than A Shot of Espresso

34. Randolph, D. D., & O'Connor, P. J. (2017). 'Stair walking is more energizing than low dose caffeine in sleep deprived young women.' Physiology & Behavior, 174, 128-135. <https://doi.org/10.1016/j.physbeh.2017.03.013>.

Yes, Walking Counts

35. Patel AV, Hildebrand JS, Leach CR, Campbell PT, Doyle C, Shuval K, Wang Y, Gapstur SM. 'Walking in Relation to Mortality in a Large Prospective Cohort of Older U.S. Adults'. Am J Prev Med. 2018 Jan;54(1):10-19. doi: 10.1016/j.amepre.2017.08.019. Epub 2017 Oct 19. PMID: 29056372.

36. JoAnn E. Manson, M.D., Dr.P.H., Philip Greenland, M.D., Andrea Z. LaCroix, Ph.D., Marcia L. Stefanick, Ph.D., Charles P. Mouton, M.D., Albert Oberman, M.D., M.P.H., Michael G. Perri, Ph.D., David S. Sheps, M.D., Mary B. Pettinger, M.S., and David S. Siscovick, M.D., M.P.H., 'Walking Compared with Vigorous Exercise for the Prevention of Cardiovascular Events in Women,' September 5, 2002, N Engl J Med 2002; 347:716-725, DOI: 10.1056/NEJMoa021067. <https://www.nejm.org/doi/full/10.1056/NEJMoa021067>.

37. Crum AJ, Langer EJ. 'Mind-set matters: exercise and the placebo effect.' Psychol Sci. 2007 Feb;18(2):165-71. doi: 10.1111/j.1467-9280.2007.01867.x. PMID: 17425538.

Biological vs. Chronological Age and Telo-Whats?

38. López-Otín C, Blasco MA, Partridge L, Serrano M, Kroemer G. 'Hallmarks of aging: An expanding universe'. Cell. 2023 Jan 19;186(2):243-278. doi: 10.1016/j.cell.2022.11.001. Epub 2023 Jan 3. PMID: 36599349.

39. Larry A. Tucker, 2020, 'Walking and biologic aging: Evidence based on NHANES telomere data', Journal of Sports Sciences, 38:9, 1026-1035, DOI: 10.1080/02640414.2020.1739896.

40. Paddy C. Dempsey, Crispin Musicha, Alex V. Rowlands, Melanie Davies, Kamlesh Khunti, Cameron Razieh, Iain Timmins, Francesco Zaccardi, Veryan Codd, Christopher P. Nelson, Tom Yates, Nilesh J. Samani. 'Investigation of a UK biobank cohort reveals causal associations of self-reported walking pace with telomere length'. Communications Biology, 2022; 5 (1) DOI: 10.1038/s42003-022-03323-x.

Heart Health

41. May 15, 2023, Heart Disease Facts, Centers for Disease Control and Prevention, <https://www.cdc.gov/heartdisease/facts.htm>.

42. Morris JN, Heady JA, Raffle PA, Roberts CG, Parks JW. 'Coronary heart-disease and physical activity of work'. Lancet. 1953 Nov 21;262(6795):1053-1057. doi: 10.1016/s0140-6736(53)90665-5. PMID: 13110049.

Walking and Cancer ... Before, During, and After

43. Patel AV, Friedenreich CM, Moore SC, Hayes SC, Silver JK, Campbell KL, Winters-Stone K, Gerber LH, George SM, Fulton JE, Denlinger C, Morris GS, Hue T, Schmitz KH, Matthews CE. 'American College of Sports Medicine Roundtable Report on Physical Activity, Sedentary Behavior, and Cancer Prevention and Control'. Med Sci Sports Exerc. 2019 Nov;51(11):2391-2402. doi: 10.1249/MSS.0000000000002117. PMID: 31626056; PMCID: PMC6814265.

44. Charles E. Matthews, Steven C. Moore, Hannah Arem, Michael B. Cook, Britton Trabert, Niclas Håkansson, Susanna C. Larsson, Alicja Wolk, Susan M. Gapstur, Brigid M. Lynch, Roger L. Milne, Neal D. Freedman, Wen-Yi Huang, Amy Berrington de Gonzalez, Cari M. Kitahara, Martha S. Linet, Eric J. Shiroma, Sven Sandin, Alpa V. Patel, and I-Min Lee. 'Amount and Intensity of Leisure-Time Physical Activity and Lower Cancer Risk,' Journal of Clinical Oncology, 2020 38:7, 686-697.

45. '5 Surprising Benefits of Walking', Harvard Health Publishing, August 25, 2022, <https://www.health.harvard.edu/staying-healthy/5-surprising-benefits-of-walking>.

46. Rebecca D. Kehm, Jeanine M. Genkinger; Robert J. MacInnis; Esther M. John, et al., 'Recreational Physical Activity Is Associated with Reduced Breast Cancer Risk in Adult Women at High Risk for Breast Cancer: A Cohort Study of Women Selected for Familial and Genetic Risk',

Population and Prevention Science, January 3 2020, <https://aacrjournals. org/cancerres/article/80/1/116/640695/Recreational-Physical-Activity-Is-Associated-with>.

47. Cannioto RA, Hutson A, Dighe S, McCann W, McCann SE, Zirpoli GR, Barlow W, Kelly KM, DeNysschen CA, Hershman DL, Unger JM, Moore HCF, Stewart JA, Isaacs C, Hobday TJ, Salim M, Hortobagyi GN, Gralow JR, Albain KS, Budd GT, Ambrosone CB. 'Physical Activity Before, During, and After Chemotherapy for High-Risk Breast Cancer: Relationships With Survival.' J National Cancer Institute. 2021 Jan 4;113(1):54-63. doi: 10.1093/jnci/djaa046. PMID: 32239145; PMCID: PMC7781460.

Sugar Rush: Walking and Diabetes

48. Khan MAB, Hashim MJ, King JK, Govender RD, Mustafa H, Al Kaabi J. 'Epidemiology of Type 2 Diabetes - Global Burden of Disease and Forecasted Trends.' J Epidemiol Glob Health. 2020 Mar;10(1):107-111. doi: 10.2991/jegh.k.191028.001. PMID: 32175717; PMCID: PMC7310804.

49. 'Diabetes: Key Facts,' World Health Organization, April 5, 2023, <https://www.who.int/news-room/fact-sheets/detail/diabetes>.

50. Ruth S. Weinstock, MD, PhD, 'Treating Type 2 Diabetes Mellitus: A Growing Epidemic', Mayo Clinic Proceedings, Volume 78, Issue 4, April 2003, DOI:https://doi.org/10.4065/78.4.411<https://www.mayo clinicproceedings.org/article/S0025-6196(11)62819-X/fulltext>.

51. Diabetes Prevention Program Research Group, 'Reduction in the Incidence of Type 2 Diabetes with Lifestyle Intervention or Metformin', February 7, 2002, N Engl J Med 2002; 346:393-403, DOI: 10.1056/NEJMoa012512. <https://www.nejm.org/doi/full/10.1056/NEJMoa012512>.

52. Loretta Dipietro, Andrei Gribok, Michelle Stevens, Larry F. Hamm, William Rumpler, 'Three 15-min Bouts of Moderate Postmeal Walking Significantly Improves 24-h Glycemic Control in Older People at Risk for Impaired Glucose Tolerance,' Diabetes Care, Volume 36, October 2013, <https://care.diabetesjournals.org/content/diacare/early/2013/06/03/dc13-0084.full.pdf>.

Lose Weight

53. Slentz CA, Duscha BD, Johnson JL, et al. 'Effects of the Amount of Exercise on Body Weight, Body Composition, and Measures of Central Obesity: STRRIDE—A Randomized Controlled Study'. Arch Intern Med. 2004;164(1):31–39. doi:10.1001/archinte.164.1.31 <https://jamanetwork.com/journals/jamainternalmedicine/fullarticle/216495>.

54. Kindel T, Martin E, Hungness E, Nagle, 'A. High failure rate of the laparoscopic-adjustable gastric band as a primary bariatric procedure.' Surg Obes Relat Dis. 2014 Nov-Dec;10(6):1070-5. doi: 10.1016/j.soard.2013.11.014. Epub 2013 Dec 6. PMID: 24630503, <https://pubmed.ncbi.nlm.nih.gov/24630503/.>.

Eat Less Chocolate

55. Taylor AH, Oliver A. 'Acute effects of brisk walking on urges to eat chocolate, affect, and responses to a stressor and chocolate cue: An experimental study.' Appetite. 2009;52: 155–60. 10.1016/j.appet.2008.09.004. <https://www.sciencedirect.com/science/article/abs/pii/S0195666308005564?via%3Dihub>.

56. Ledochowski L, Ruedl G, Taylor AH, Kopp M (2015) 'Acute Effects of Brisk Walking on Sugary Snack Cravings in Overweight People, Affect and Responses to a Manipulated Stress Situation and to a Sugary Snack Cue: A Crossover Study'. PLoS ONE 10(3): e0119278. <https://doi.org/10.1371/journal.pone.0119278>.

57. Taylor A, Katomeri M. 'Walking reduces cue-elicited cigarette cravings and withdrawal symptoms, and delays ad libitum smoking'. Nicotine Tob Res. 2007 Nov;9(11):1183-90. doi: 10.1080/14622200701648896. PMID: 17978993.

58. Ussher M, Nunziata P, Cropley M, West R., 'Effect of a short bout of exercise on tobacco withdrawal symptoms and desire to smoke.' Psychopharmacology (Berl). 2001 Oct;158(1):66-72. doi: 10.1007/s002130100846.

Oh My Aching Back: Walking and Back Pain

59. Ekalak Sitthipornvorakul, Thaniya Klinsophon, Rattaporn Sihawong, Prawit Janwantanakul, 'The effects of walking intervention in patients with chronic low back pain: A meta-analysis of randomized controlled trials,' Musculoskeletal Science and Practice, Volume 34, 2018, Pages 38-46, ISSN 2468-7812,

60. Sitthipornvorakul, E., Klinsophon, T., Sihawong, R., & Janwantanakul, P. (2018). 'The effects of walking intervention in patients with chronic low back pain: A meta-analysis of randomized controlled trials'. Musculoskeletal Science and Practice, 34, 38-46. <https://doi.org/10.1016/j.msksp.2017.12.003>.

Oh My Aching Knees: Walking and Arthritis

61. 'Arthritis,' Centers for Disease Control and Prevention, November 3, 2021, <https://www.cdc.gov/chronicdisease/resources/publications/factsheets/arthritis.htm>.

62. Mayo Clinic Staff, 'Exercise Helps East Arthritis Pain and Stiffness,' <https://www.mayoclinic.org/diseases-conditions/arthritis/in-depth/arthritis/art-20047971.>

63. Lo, G.H., Vinod, S., Richard, M.J., Harkey, M.S., McAlindon, T.E., Kriska, A.M., Rockette-Wagner, B., Eaton, C.B., Hochberg, M.C., Jackson, R.D., Kwoh, C.K., Nevitt, M.C. and Driban, J.B. (2022), 'Association Between Walking for Exercise and Symptomatic and Structural Progression in Individuals With Knee Osteoarthritis: Data From the Osteoarthritis Initiative Cohort.' Arthritis Rheumatol, 74: 1660-1667. <https://doi.org/10.1002/art.42241>.

Stronger Bones

64. Lan YS, Feng YJ. 'The volume of brisk walking is the key determinant of BMD improvement in premenopausal women.' PLoS One. 2022 March 16;17(3):e0265250. doi: 10.1371/journal.pone.0265250.

65. Benedetti MG, Furlini G, Zati A, Letizia Mauro G., 'The Effectiveness of Physical Exercise on Bone Density in Osteoporotic Patients.' Biomed Res Int. 2018 Dec 23;2018:4840531. doi: 10.1155/2018/4840531. PMID: 30671455; PMCID: PMC6323511.

66. Krall EA, Dawson-Hughes B., 'Walking is related to bone density and rates of bone loss.' Am J Med. 1994 Jan;96(1):20-6. doi: 10.1016/0002-9343(94)90111-2. PMID: 8304358. <https://pubmed.ncbi.nlm.nih.gov/8304358/>.

67. Bone Health and Osteoporosis Foundation, Just for Men, <https://www.bonehealthandosteoporosis.org/preventing-fractures/general-facts/just-for-men/>.

Better Balance

68. Hall, K. S., Cohen, H. J., Pieper, C. F., Fillenbaum, G. G., Kraus, W. E., Huffman, K. M., Cornish, M. A., Shiloh, A., Flynn, C., Sloane, R., Newby, L. K., & Morey, M. C. (2017). 'Physical Performance Across the Adult Life Span: Correlates With Age and Physical Activity'. The Journals of Gerontology: Series A, 72(4), 572-578. https://doi.org/10.1093/gerona/glw120 <https://academic.oup.com/biomedgerontology/article/72/4/572/2629941>.

69. Centers for Disease Control and Prevention, 'Keep on Your Feet – Preventing Older Adult Falls', March 24, 2023, <https://www.cdc.gov/injury/features/older-adult-falls/index.html>.

70. Okubo Y, Osuka Y, Jung S, Rafael F, Tsujimoto T, Aiba T, Kim T, Tanaka K. 'Walking can be more effective than balance training in fall prevention among community-dwelling older adults.' Geriatr Gerontol Int. 2016 Jan;16(1):118-25. doi: 10.1111/ggi.12444. Epub 2015 Jan 22. PMID: 25613322 <https://pubmed.ncbi.nlm.nih.gov/25613322/>.

Menopause is Sneaky. Walking Helps.

71. Javadivala Z, Allahverdipour H, Asghari Jafarabadi M, Emami A. 'An Interventional strategy of physical activity promotion for reduction of menopause symptoms'. Health Promot Perspect. 2020 Nov 7;10(4):383-392. doi: 10.34172/hpp.2020.57. PMID: 33312934; PMCID: PMC7722991.

Get Sick Less

72. Ikeda T, Inoue S, Konta T, et al. 'Can Daily Walking Alone Reduce Pneumonia-Related Mortality among Older People?' Scientific Reports. 2020

May;10(1):8556. DOI: 10.1038/s41598-020-65440-z. PMID: 32444618; PMCID: PMC7244731.

73. Nieman DC, Wentz LM. 'The compelling link between physical activity and the body's defense system.' J Sport Health Sci. 2019 May;8(3):201-217. doi: 10.1016/j.jshs.2018.09.009. Epub 2018 Nov 16. PMID: 31193280; PMCID: PMC6523821.<https://www.ncbi.nlm.nih.gov/pmc/articles/PMC6523821/>.

74. Sand KL, Flatebo T, Andersen MB, Maghazachi AA. 'Effects of exercise on leukocytosis and blood hemostasis in 800 healthy young females and males.' World J Exp Med. 2013 Feb 20;3(1):11-20. doi: 10.5493/wjem.v3.i1.11. PMID: 24520541; PMCID: PMC3905589.

Protect Your Peepers

75. Tseng VL, Yu F, Coleman AL. 'Association between Exercise Intensity and Glaucoma in the National Health and Nutrition Examination Survey.' Ophthalmol Glaucoma. 2020 Sep-Oct;3(5):393-402. doi: 10.1016/j.ogla.2020.06.001. Epub 2020 Jun 7. PMID: 32741639;

76. Lee, Moon Jeong; Wang, Jiangxia; Friedman, David S.; Boland, Michael V.; De Moraes, Carlos G.; Ramulu, Pradeep Y. (2018). 'Greater Physical Activity Is Associated with Slower Visual Field Loss in Glaucoma.' Ophthalmology, S0161642018307929–. doi:10.1016/j.ophtha.2018.10.012.

But Wait, Is It Exercise That Helps or Do Healthier People Just Move More?

77. Kujala UM, Kaprio J, Sarna S, Koskenvuo M. 'Relationship of leisure-time physical activity and mortality: the Finnish twin cohort.' JAMA. 1998 Feb 11;279(6):440-4. doi: 10.1001/jama.279.6.440. PMID: 9466636.

Benefits of Barefoot

78. Wearing SC, Reed L, Hooper SL, Bartold S, Smeathers JE, Brauner T. 'Running shoes increase achilles tendon load in walking: an acoustic propagation study.' Med Sci Sports Exerc. 2014 Aug;46(8):1604-9. doi: 10.1249/MSS.0000000000000256. PMID: 24500535.

79. Oschman JL, Chevalier G, Brown R. 'The effects of grounding (earthing) on inflammation, the immune response, wound healing, and prevention and treatment of chronic inflammatory and autoimmune diseases.' J Inflamm Res. 2015 Mar 24;8:83-96. doi: 10.2147/JIR.S69656. PMID: 25848315; PMCID: PMC4378297.

That Said . . .

80. I-Min Lee, MBBS, ScD; Eric J. Shiroma, ScD; Masamitsu Kamada, PhD; et al David R. Bassett, PhD; Charles E. Matthews, PhD; Julie E. Buring, ScD, 'Association of Step Volume and Intensity With All-Cause Mortality in Older Women,' JAMA Intern Med. 2019;179(8):1105-1112. doi:10.1001/jamainternmed.2019.0899.

81. Amanda E Paluch, PhD, Shivangi Bajpai, MS, Prof David R Bassett, PhD, Prof Mercedes, R Carnethon, PhD, Prof Ulf Ekelund, PhD, Prof Kelly R Evenson, PhD, et al. 'Daily steps and all-cause mortality: a meta-analysis of 15 international cohorts,' The Lancet, Volume 7, Issue 3, March 2022, DOI:https://doi.org/10.1016/S2468-2667(21)00302-9, <https://www.thelancet.com/journals/lanpub/article/PIIS2468-2667(21)00302-9/fulltext>.

82. Master, H., Annis, J., Huang, S. et al. 'Association of step counts over time with the risk of chronic disease in the All of Us Research Program.' Nature Medicine 28, 2301–2308 (2022). <https://doi.org/10.1038/s41591-022-02012-w>.

83. 'Step up your walking game. The life-extending effects of a daily walk.' Harvard Health Publishing, Harvard Medical School. June 21, 2021. <https://www.health.harvard.edu/heart-health/step-up-your-walking-game>.

Benefits of a 10-Minute Walk

84. Jakicic, John M.1; Kraus, William E.2; Powell, Kenneth E.3; Campbell, Wayne W.4; Janz, Kathleen F.5; Troiano, Richard P.6; Sprow, Kyle6; Torres, Andrea; Piercy, Katrina. 'Association between Bout Duration of Physical Activity and Health: Systematic Review.' Medicine & Science in Sports & Exercise 51(6):p 1213-1219, June 2019. | DOI: 10.1249/MSS.0000000000001933.

85. Murphy MH, Lahart I, Carlin A, Murtagh E., 'The Effects of Continuous Compared to Accumulated Exercise on Health: A Meta-Analytic Review.' Sports Medicine 2019 Oct;49(10):1585-1607. doi: 10.1007/s40279-019-01145-2. PMID: 31267483; PMCID: PMC6745307.

86. Bhammar, Dharini, Angadi, Siddhartha, Gaesser, Glenn, 'Effects of Frac-tionized and Continuous Exercise on 24-h Ambulatory Blood Pressure.' Medicine & Science in Sports & Exercise 44(12):p 2270-2276, December 2012. | DOI: 10.1249/MSS.0b013e3182663117

87. Anxiety and Depression Association of America, 'Exercise for Stress and Anxiety,' <https://adaa.org/living-with-anxiety/managing-anxiety/exercise-stress-and-anxiety>.

88. Buffey, A.J., Herring, M.P., Langley, C.K. et al. 'The Acute Effects of Interrupting Prolonged Sitting Time in Adults with Standing and Light-Intensity Walking on Biomarkers of Cardiometabolic Health in Adults: A Systematic Review and Meta-analysis'. Sports Med 52, 1765–1787 (2022). <https://doi.org/10.1007/s40279-022-01649-4>.

89. Saint-Maurice PF, Graubard BI, Troiano RP, Berrigan D, Galuska DA, Fulton JE, Matthews CE., 'Estimated Number of Deaths Prevented Through Increased Physical Activity Among US Adults.' JAMA Intern Med. 2022 Mar 1;182(3):349-352. doi: 10.1001/jamainternmed.2021.7755. PMID: 35072698; PMCID: PMC8787676.

When To Walk?

90. Schumacher LM, Thomas JG, Raynor HA, Rhodes RE, Bond DS. 'Consistent Morning Exercise May Be Beneficial for Individuals With Obesity.' Exercise Sport Science Rev. 2020 Oct;48(4):201-208. doi: 10.1249/JES.0000000000000226. PMID: 32658039; PMCID: PMC7492403.

91. Mead MN. 'Benefits of sunlight: a bright spot for human health.' Environ Health Perspect. 2008 Apr;116(4):A160-7. doi: 10.1289/ehp.116-a160. Erratum in: Environ Health Perspect. 2008 May;116(5):A197. PMID: 18414615; PMCID: PMC2290997. <https://www.ncbi.nlm.nih.gov/pmc/articles/PMC2290997/>.

92. Colberg SR, Zarrabi L, Bennington L, Nakave A, Thomas Somma C, Swain DP, Sechrist SR. 'Postprandial walking is better for lowering the glycemic effect of dinner than pre-dinner exercise in type 2 diabetic individuals.' J Am Med Dir Assoc. 2009 Jul;10(6):394-7. doi: 10.1016/j.jamda.2009.03.015. Epub 2009 May 21. PMID: 19560716.

93. Shambrook P, Kingsley MI, Taylor NF, Wundersitz DW, Wundersitz CE, Paton CD, Gordon BA. 'A comparison of acute glycaemic responses to accumulated or single bout walking exercise in apparently healthy, insufficiently active adults.' J Sci Med Sport. 2020 Oct; 23(10):902-907. doi: 10.1016/j.jsams.2020.02.015. Epub 2020 Mar 6. PMID: 32173259.

94. Loretta DiPietro, Andrei Gribok, Michelle S. Stevens, Larry F. Hamm, William Rumpler, 'Three 15-min Bouts of Moderate Postmeal Walking Significantly Improves 24-h Glycemic Control in Older People at Risk for Impaired Glucose Tolerance'. Diabetes Care 1 October 2013; 36 (10): 3262–3268. <https://doi.org/10.2337/dc13-0084>.

95. Janský L, Pospíšilová D, Honzová S, Ulicný B, Srámek P, Zeman V, Kamínková J. 'Immune system of cold-exposed and cold-adapted humans.' Eur J Appl Physiol Occup Physiol. 1996;72(5-6):445-50. doi: 10.1007/BF00242274. PMID: 8925815.

96. Blondin DP, Labbé SM, Tingelstad HC, Noll C, Kunach M, Phoenix S, Guérin B, Turcotte EE, Carpentier AC, Richard D, Haman F. 'Increased brown adipose tissue oxidative capacity in cold-acclimated humans.' J Clin Endocrinol Metab. 2014 Mar;99(3):E438-46. doi: 10.1210/jc.2013-3901. Epub 2014 Jan 13. PMID: 24423363; PMCID: PMC4213359.

97. Ikäheimo TM. 'Cardiovascular diseases, cold exposure and exercise.' Temperature (Austin). 2018 Feb 1;5(2):123-146. doi: 10.1080/23328940.2017.1414014. PMID: 30377633; PMCID: PMC6204981.

The Joy of Flanerie

98. Organisation for EconomicCo-operation and Development, <https://stats.oecd.org/index.aspx?DataSetCode=ANHRS>.

Walking as Meditation

99. Thich Nhat Hanh 2005 Call me by My True Names – The Collected Poems of Thich Nhat Hanh, Parallax Press.

Then, Set Your Own Goal

100. Patel MS, Bachireddy C, Small DS, et al. 'Effect of Goal-Setting Approaches Within a Gamification Intervention to Increase Physical Activity Among Economically Disadvantaged Adults at Elevated Risk for Major Adverse Cardiovascular Events: The ENGAGE Randomized Clinical Trial.' JAMA Cardiol. 2021;6(12):1387–1396. doi:10.1001/jamacardio.2021.3176 <https://jamanetwork.com/journals/jamacardiology/article-abstract/2783498>.

Two Ways to Keep Going: Build a Walking Habit. Or Don't.

101. Duhigg, Charles 2012. The Power of Habit. Why We Do What We Do in Life and Business. Random House.

Find a Friend, Or Five

102. Christian H, Bauman A, Epping JN, Levine GN, McCormack G, Rhodes RE, Richards E, Rock M, Westgarth C. 'Encouraging Dog Walking for Health Promotion and Disease Prevention.' Am J Lifestyle Med. 2016 Apr 17;12(3):233-243. doi: 10.1177/1559827616643686. PMID: 30202393; PMCID: PMC6124971.

103. Westgarth, C., Christley, R.M., Jewell, C. et al. 'Dog owners are more likely to meet physical activity guidelines than people without a dog: An investigation of the association between dog ownership and physical activity levels in a UK community.' Sci Rep 9, 5704 (2019). <https://doi.org/10.1038/s41598-019-41254-6>.

Walking as an Antidote to the Loneliness Epidemic

104. Richard Weissbourd, Milena Batanova, Virginia Lovison, and Eric Torres, 'Loneliness in America How the Pandemic Has Deepened an Epidemic of Loneliness and What We Can Do About It' Harvard Graduate School of Education, Making Caring Common Project <https://static1.squarespace.com/static/5b7c56e255b02c683659fe43/t/6021776bdd04957c4557c212/1612805995893/Loneliness+in+America+2021_02_08_FINAL.pdf>.

105. Demarinis S. 'Loneliness at epidemic levels in America.' Explore (NY). 2020 Sep-Oct;16(5):278-279. doi: 10.1016/j.explore.2020.06.008. Epub 2020 Jun 28. PMID: 32674944; PMCID: PMC7321652.

106. Dr. Vivek Murthy, 'Work and the Loneliness Epidemic,' Harvard Business Review, September 26, 2017 <https://hbr.org/2017/09/work-and-the-loneliness-epidemic>.

Shared Experiences

107. Boothby EJ, Clark MS, Bargh JA., 'Shared experiences are amplified.' Psychol Sci. 2014 Dec;25(12):2209-16. doi: 10.1177/0956797614551162. Epub 2014 Oct 1. PMID: 25274583. <https://clarkrelationshiplab.yale.edu/sites/default/files/files/BoothbyClarkBargh(1).pdf>.

Undistracted Time

108. Przybylski, A. K., & Weinstein, N. (2013). 'Can you connect with me now? How the presence of mobile communication technology influences face-to-face conversation quality.' Journal of Social and Personal Relationships, 30(3), 237–246. <https://doi.org/10.1177/0265407512453827>.

109. Roberts, J. A., & David, M. E. (2016). 'My life has become a major distraction from my cell phone: Partner phubbing and relationship satisfaction among romantic partners'. Computers in Human Behavior, 54, 134-141. <https://doi.org/10.1016/j.chb.2015.07.058>.

Synchronicity

110. Zivotofsky, A.Z., Hausdorff, J.M. 'The sensory feedback mechanisms enabling couples to walk synchronously: An initial investigation'. J NeuroEngineering Rehabil 4, 28 (2007). <https://doi.org/10.1186/1743-0003-4-28>.

111. Bazhydai M, Ke H, Thomas H, Wong MKY, Westermann G. 'Investigating the effect of synchronized movement on toddlers' word learning'. Front Psychol. 2022 Nov 24;13:1008404. doi: 10.3389/fpsyg.2022.1008404. PMID: 36506988; PMCID: PMC9731293.

Walking with Your Partner: Jennifer's Story

112. Yorgason, Jeremy B.; Johnson, Lee N.; Hill, Melanie S.; Selland, Bailey (2018). 'Marital Benefits of Daily Individual and Conjoint Exercise Among Older Couples'. Family Relations, 67(2), 227–239. doi:10.1111/fare.12307. Notably, this study has several limitations including the absence of any couples of color or same-sex. Nevertheless, it is one of the few studies that has looked at the specific impact of joint exercise on marital satisfaction.

Don't Look Them In the Eyes: Walking with Your Teen

113. 'New Red Robin Survey Reveals 73% of Children Wish They Had More Time to Connect With Their Family' Red Robin Restaurants', Cision PR Newswire, 24 Jul. 2019, <https://www.prnewswire.com/news-releases/new-red-robin-survey-reveals-73-of-children-wish-they-had-more-time-to-connect-with-their-family-300889904.html>.

Wanna' Go for a Walk and Fight? Walking and Conflict Resolution.

114. Webb, C. E., Rossignac-Milon, M., & Higgins, E. T. (2017). 'Stepping forward together: Could walking facilitate interpersonal conflict resolution?' American Psychologist, 72(4), 374–385. <https://doi.org/10.1037/a0040431>.

Benefits of Walkable Communities

115. Project for Public Spaces, PBS, Jan. 3 2010 <https://www.pps.org/article/wwhyte>.

116. Leyden KM. 'Social capital and the built environment: the importance of walkable neighborhoods.' Am J Public Health. 2003 Sep; 93(9):1546-51. doi: 10.2105/ajph.93.9.1546. PMID: 12948978; PMCID: PMC1448008.

The Power of Walking Groups

117. Hanson S, Jones A. 'Is there evidence that walking groups have health benefits? A systematic review and meta-analysis.' Br J Sports Med. 2015 Jun;49(11):710-5. doi: 10.1136/bjsports-2014-094157. Epub 2015 Jan 19. PMID: 25601182; PMCID: PMC4453623.

When You Need it Most, You Will Feel Like it Least

118. Boris Cheval, Eda Tipura, Nicolas Burra, Jaromil Frossard, Julien Chanal, Dan Orsholits, Rémi Radel, Matthieu P. Boisgontier, 'Avoiding sedentary behaviors requires more cortical resources than avoiding physical activity: An EEG study,' Neuropsychologia, Volume 119, 2018, Pages 68-80, ISSN 0028-3932, <https://doi.org/10.1016/j.neuropsychologia.2018.07.029.>.

Acknowledgements

This is the book that almost wasn't. And wouldn't be if not for the stalwart support of a few people who believed in me and believed in this project.

Eric, not only are you a rock of love and support, but by example, you have taught me more about grit than anyone or anything. I owe all of the wonderful things in my life to you.

To my mom, who has always been my first reader and who has always encouraged me to keep going. Thank you for your insights, your edits, and the moments when you push me to make the writing better.

To my dad, who we lost just months before this book was published. My heart breaks to know that you won't read all that you inspired in this book and in my life, which is, pretty much, everything.

And to Maddie and Mason, it all would be nothing without you both.

About the Author

Joyce Shulman is a serial entrepreneur, idea junkie, addicted skier, sometimes CrossFitter, recovering attorney, and author. But mostly, she is a joyful wanderer.

As the co-founder and CEO of 99 Walks & Jetti Fitness, she helped build a multimillion-dollar company and that has helped tens of thousands discover, sustain, and level up their intentional walking practice.

A mom of two almost-adults, Joyce lives in Sag Harbor, New York, with her husband and regular canine walking companion, Moose.

www.ingramcontent.com/pod-product-compliance
Lightning Source LLC
La Vergne TN
LVHW091217080426
835509LV00009B/1048